KATHRYN JARVIS

A RED DOOR

Black Rose Writing | Texas

©2020 by Kathryn Jarvis
All rights reserved. No part of this book may be reproduced, stored in a retrieval system or transmitted in any form or by any means without the prior written permission of the publishers, except by a reviewer who may quote brief passages in a review to be printed in a newspaper, magazine or journal.

The author grants the final approval for this literary material.

First printing

This is a work of nonfiction and is based on true events. Some names have been changed to protect the identity of the individuals.

ISBN: 978-1-68433-544-2
PUBLISHED BY BLACK ROSE WRITING
www.blackrosewriting.com

Printed in the United States of America
Suggested Retail Price (SRP) $18.95

A Red Door is printed in Chaparral Pro

*As a planet-friendly publisher, Black Rose Writing does its best to eliminate unnecessary waste to reduce paper usage and energy costs, while never compromising the reading experience. As a result, the final word count vs. page count may not meet common expectations.

For Lucy and Jake

A RED DOOR

Prologue
During It All

I began this story scribbling on a yellow legal pad at the kitchen table after the kids were in bed. Sometimes, when I wrote I'd drink wine, sometimes too much, then not at all. That's probably when I was gulping Xanax to get through the days and then, even more to survive the nights. I couldn't live in the therapist's office, so I started to write short vignettes chronicling the fear, the anger and the hope. After a time, at the end of the long, difficult journey, I went back and finished the story, realizing, as I'd been told by a gifted medium, that I had balanced on the precipice, and by grace, fate, karma, and love had not fallen in.

So much happened during these early years (1988-1992, in my case) as we dealt with the specter and stigma of AIDS, most of it tragic and frightening, but like many things in this balance of life, there was evidence of goodness and courage; people with AIDS, family and friends who championed them, and even those who were frightened, yet moved past their fears because of love and commitment. I've been accused of being a Pollyanna, and I graciously accept that accusation. Call it resilience, grit, faith or Pollyanna, you get out of bed, wash your face, and marvel that your body can take in breath. Then you say thank you, smile and salute the sun.

Chapter 1
The Beginning

In my position at a newly established college, I traveled more than I had in the past. We were out there, doing presentations, sharing our current research, marketing and working it all over the country. It was glamorous at first, but I had quickly tired of the plane rides, schmoozing and leaving my young children. My husband was a good Dad, but even super dads were challenged by two small kids under six years.

On the west coast, I was three hours behind the cocktail hour at home, when no amount of alcohol was sufficient, you still had to function, reasonable demands were dashed and all that mattered was getting some form of food into fussy little mouths.

I picked up the phone. Smiling, I pictured my young daughter's Campbell soup cheeks and bright blue eyes as I listened to her pent up excitement rushing through the long distance lines. With great import, she outlined the latest household drama that had occurred since I had been away, 'Daddy didn't suck the bat up in the vacuum like you did. He scooted it out with a broom.' I assured her that my poor bat was most likely sick cause it knocked itself out on the chandelier before I sucked it up.

In the background, I could hear a chuckle from my husband, Mark as he came on the phone reminding me that if the bat wasn't dead, it surely was after I'd duct taped it shut in the hose. That vacuum didn't get used for at least a month until I was sure it wouldn't come out and get me. It had provided a good excuse not to vacuum.

Not wanting to be left out of the conversation, Lucy hurriedly injected, that her little brother, Jake was a scaredy cat and he ran in the kitchen, but she helped.

"That you did, brave girl. Now run get Jake so he can talk to Mommy. She's on long distance," my husband added.

With a dramatic sigh, Lucy relented. "Bye mommy, love you," and banged down the extension.

"You too," I gave up to the air. "Well, she seems to be getting along just fine. How are y'all? I miss you."

"Oh, we're okay. We miss you too and let me say, tomorrow can come none too soon."

"Has it been rough?"

"No, not really. I'm just tired."

"Is this my Mommy?" a child's small voice echoed through the phone.

"Yes, dear boy, it's Mommy."

"Are you still far away?" Jake asked.

"I am. I'm all the way across the whole United States, but I'll be home tomorrow. You and Lucy and Daddy are picking me up at the big airport."

"Daddy says we can ride the up high trains and get McDonald's."

"That is special! That's two treats and then, you never know what Mommy might bring."

"A big bike?"

"Not this time angel. Maybe, later."

"When I'm five?"

"Could be. Now let me talk to Daddy and give yourself a big hug and kiss from me."

I laughed when a loud kissing noise sounded in my ear. "You there?"

Mark answered, with a chuckle. "Yeah, I had to help him hug."

"He's a hoot. Anyway, I'll be in late tomorrow afternoon if the plane's on time."

"And we'll be there. I'll do my best to keep them somewhat contained and my dear, enjoy your last night of freedom. Do something wild like enjoy a meal without interruptions."

I grinned at the reminder of dinner chaos. "I don't know what to do without at least one spilling of something. I sort of just sit and stare, but, I'll be back to help control the madness soon." I added, "I love you."

"Me too."

"Well, tell Lucy bye and give her kisses from me." I waited a moment listening to Mark's soft breathing, "One more thing. How's your neck?"

"Oh, the lump's still there. No pain. Just annoying. We'll have plenty of time to talk when you get home. Don't worry. I'm fine, really."

"I'll let it alone for now, but you know…"

"I know. The operative word is 'for now'." He continued, "And I promise to call the doctor in the morning. I know you won't let up. It's one of your endearing qualities, sweetheart."

"And you wouldn't want me any other way."

"That is true."

"So, I'll see you tomorrow then."

"Yes. Bye, love."

"Good night."

I had been concerned about my husband for a while now. Never sick, he always had incredible energy and now this swollen gland on his neck and a cold that had lingered for weeks. And even before he started feeling lousy, our sex life had all but gone away. We'd ignored it because it had been a non-issue; we were both exhausted, with two young children and work. Lucy was not quite two when Jake was born, and neither of us wanted another child anytime soon. With a young child and baby to care for, sex had become less important. Frankly, I looked forward to bedtime when I gratefully collapsed. Now that Jake was older and Lucy starting to fend for herself, I realized our sex life ceased to exist. We talked about it, made plans to go away, and even then, Mark slept most of the time. I'd been angry, but figured he was worn out from work and needed the rest.

The anger buried, it resurfaced as frustration when I remembered how hot sex used to be. We had made love all over town. Once, purposely stuck in the elevator; another time clutched in the corner, tucked away in the back of Bloomingdale's and a long while ago, tossing around on the sailboat while the storms raged. It was not like Mark to be sick. He was the one all our friends voted to be with on the lifeboat. He'd slay the sharks, live for days on shark blood, get us all home safely and joke about our envious tans. He will have an appointment with the doctor by the time I got home. He promised.

Back in my room after a quiet supper at the bar, I gazed out at the twinkling lights in the distant mountains. Being away for almost a week, I thought I'd feel rested. Instead, I was tired, too. Unsettling dreams had kept me up. Always hopeful, maybe tonight I'd sleep.

I drifted off and then the dream hurtled me into the acrid smoke and the stench from the pyres piled high with dead bodies. My eyes stinging, I stumbled and slipped, sliding down toward the roaring river, always waking up before I hit the frigid water.

My feet hit the carpeted floor. I staggered into the bathroom, turned on the faucet and splashed cold water on my face. Flipping on the overhead light I peered into the harsh fluorescence of the bathroom mirror, tracing the smile lines around my mouth, all those years of baby oil and iodine baking on Florida beaches. And, that gap in my front teeth. I should have had braces, and if only my boobs were bigger, my stomach flatter, the freckles fewer and were women ever satisfied with our bodies?

The luminous clock on the bedside table read 5:00 am, Pacific time. It was eight o'clock on the east coast, and Mark would be getting the kids out the door, Lucy to kindergarten and Jake to nursery school. Tomorrow morning he'd have a chance to kick back, I'd be back on duty. Shrugging out of my damp nightgown, I turned on the shower and stepped in, the hot water cleansing away the remnants of the miserable dream.

Two times in my life, I regretted my long legs, the first, in sixth grade, a head taller that most of the boys, the other, now, cramped in a tiny seat on a crowded plane soaring somewhere over the Rockies. Large men on either side hemmed me in.

I closed my eyes and leaned back against the head rest. The pins that held up my messy bun jabbed into my scalp. In a fit I jerked out the large clips and thick hair tumbled down. Power dressing was overrated. One shoulder pad in my jacket had migrated to my chest giving me a third boob, the pantyhose squeezed my thighs and my bra held me like a vice. The plane was stifling. I channeled the air vent toward my face. It was well past time to get up and move about the cabin.

"Excuse me," I beamed at the man on the aisle and clambered over his knees. Navigating the narrow aisle, my head tickled the close ceiling. Once safely inside the miniscule restroom, I peeled off the stockings, tossed them down the rubbish chute, tore off my bra, and stuffed it into the jacket pocket, and readjusted the shoulder pad. Weaving my way back to the seat, I plopped down and within minutes fell into a dreamless sleep.

As the plane touched down, I woke up. At the gate, scanning the waiting throng, I heard familiar shrieking, "Mommy!" Jake boisterously bolted from Mark. I caught him up in a tight embrace.

"Oh Mommy, Mommy, I missed you so much**,**" he murmured, his face nestled in my neck.

I inhaled his little boy smells. I seemed he'd gotten taller in a few days.

Hand in hand, Jake and I walked over to Lucy and Mark. The children were so different, Lucy quiet, an observer, often a detached participant in the game of childhood, cautious and watchful before attempting anything. Mark and I had laughed that Lucy preferred tea at the Copley to Cheerios in the sandbox. Mark's shadow, she followed him everywhere, and he seemed to give her the affection that he sometimes had difficulty showing others. Kneeling down I grabbed her in a bear hug.

"Mommy, I'm so glad you're back. I missed you so much too, and Daddy wouldn't buy me a thing," she fawned a pout, "cause he said you'd bring presents."

Laughing, I looked at Mark, "Well, aren't you the original meany." I stood and kissed him.

"We're glad you're home," he said, his voice tired. "You look rested. And, different." His gaze took me in. "Your hair's down. Makes you look younger, as lovely as ever, just not as sophisticated, less professional woman on the move," he grinned, and pecked me on the cheek.

Self-consciously, I smoothed my mussed hair.

"It's not big, just an observation. Your hair's fine. Come on, let's get out of here before the rain starts." He picked up Jake and I took Lucy's hand as we went to collect my luggage.

Leaving the airport, tangled in the snarled Orlando traffic, Lucy and Jake strapped in the backseat of the car were as usual, fighting. I spun around and spoke firmly to the children, but the bickering continued.

The steady, streaming rain had started. Mark stared straight ahead, his hands glued to the steering wheel as he unsuccessfully attempted to negotiate a quicker route; a Boston driver in Florida traffic. The children's fussing continued. Finally, Mark snapped, eye balling them in the rear view mirror. "Goddammit, if the two of you don't stop it right now I'm going to stop this car and put you out in the rain."

I stared at his clean profile and furrowed brow and said nothing.

Peace briefly reined then Lucy began to whine, "Daddy look, he bit me and I'm bleeding."

Turning, I took Lucy's finger in my hand. "Let me see, I'm sure it's okay. There's no blood, it's just red." I eyeballed Jake with my meanest Mommy stare. "Do not bite your sister again or there will be NO Ninja Turtles."

"But, she hit me," he whimpered, his lower lip quivering.

Steamed, Mark erupted. "Jesus, they behave like hellions and don't listen to a word you say." His hands vise like on the steering wheel, he whipped his head around, dangerously weaving through the tangled traffic mess. "Jake and Lucy, for the last time shut up!"

I was stunned by this show of quick temper. "Mark, they're just kids and stuck in the car in the rain. What do you expect? They're not going to sit quietly while we listen to NPR."

Staring straight ahead, he snapped, "I know that. You just have no control over them."

"Was the week *that* bad?"

"No, the week was not *that* bad. It's just time they had a little discipline."

"Look, let's not do this now. It's late. I just got home. We're all tired."

A few quiet minutes went by. I looked over at Mark, "Has the lump gone down? I can't see it."

"That's because it's under my collar," reaching up he rolled down the edge of the upturned collar, the lump in his neck about the size of a large Agee.

"Did you make an appointment?"

"Yeah, the first available was late next week."

"How have you been feeling otherwise?"

"I'm okay. My stomach is bothering me but it's probably an ulcer. My dad had ulcers. Drove him crazy."

"Are you still real tired?"

"Who wouldn't be, taking care of two small terrorists?" He sighed, "God, would I love to get away for even a day or two."

"Really? You're serious. You think you can get away? You're always so busy."

"Well, yeah, but I think I can manage for a couple of days."

"You know, we could do a long weekend. No classes for me on Friday. Annie would take the kids, they're good playmates for James. If she can't, Sam might, if he's in town. I can see if the condo in Boca Grande's available."

Smiling, I put my hand on his knee, "Sleep in, sip gin and tonics, lie in the sun and maybe, even make love." I raised my eyebrows, "Remember that?"

"Getting away would be a good thing," his voice trailed off when a loud wail followed by a slap came from the back seat.

I whirled around, "If you don't stop it NOW there will be no treats! Look, there's a car with one light, Popeye! See how many we can find. Lulu you count and Jake say when you see one."

The enforced truce continued and soon we arrived home.

After tucking the children in, I made arrangements for the upcoming weekend, called Annie about the kids and then reserved the condo for Friday till Sunday. Mark was in bed when I came into the room.

"All done. We have the condo and Annie will come stay with the kids."

"Great," he mumbled and rolled over shutting his eyes.

His lack of interest dampened my spirits, but once I climbed into bed I fell asleep.

The week sped by. The lump on Mark's neck grew more visible so he kept his collar pulled up. We dropped the children off at school, and by afternoon sped south on route 75. As we crossed over the salt water marshes, I rolled down the window, took in a deep breath, inhaling the earthy smells and luxuriating in the feel of the damp air on my face. A native New Englander, Mark vacillated between indifference and dislike of the humidity and turned up the air conditioning in the car.

By the time, we reached the island, the first stars were lighting up the night sky, the Milky Way a dusting of fine powder scattered across the grey blue. The gentle sound of the surf slapping the mangroves played outside the screen porch as we sat chatting and sipping gin and tonics. When he finished his drink, Mark got up and headed for bed. I sat in the quiet, listening to the night sounds in the nearby marsh and then went into the bedroom.

Mark was in the bathroom as I slipped on the slinky silk nightgown he had given me last year for Valentine's. "When you're through, let me know."

"I'm done."

I brushed my teeth and washed my face, and when I came out of the bathroom Mark was propped up in the king sized bed, his eyes shut. Climbing in, I edged close to him, gliding my hand over his chest. I snuggled into his arms.

He hugged me close, admiring my nightgown. I reached up and kissed him deeply on the mouth.

"Honey, I'm exhausted."

Surprised, I stopped before the heated words tumbled out. Maybe he's really sick. Maybe it's me. And it was a drive. I brushed my lips over his stubbly cheek and rolled over, falling into a troubled sleep.

The next night repeated the same pattern. I was annoyed, and reminded Mark that one of the reasons we'd gone away was to make love without kids. Mark made no excuses, but confessed he was worried about the lump.

"I'm sorry." I touched his shoulder, "I wasn't thinking. It's just that you seemed okay today, sailing. I miss making love with you and I had hoped," my voice fading off, troubled. "Mark, I'm worried too, but it will be all right. I thought maybe sex would take your mind off it."

"It won't. I'm really preoccupied with this, and I'll feel better when I know what it is." He hugged me close. "You understand that."

"Of course, I do. I'm sorry."

"No need for sorry. I just need some sleep."

Mark was out in a few minutes, gently breathing.

I lay awake brooding beside him, finally closed my eyes and drifted into a worrisome slumber.

Chapter 2

Anxiously waiting, I sat in the lackluster waiting room of the surgeon's office, and idly thumbed through the dog-eared magazines, the glossy photos a shiny blur. Usually, I was amused by the mindless nonsense and devoured tabloid stories as a welcome escape from reality, but today even the latest who was cheating on whom held no interest. I tossed the magazine on the cluttered table and went over to where the mud black coffee was stewing. I didn't want coffee, just needed something to do with my hands.

I crossed to the reception desk, and told the woman with the puffy hair and thin lips I would be outside. She glanced up without speaking. The other woman continued talking on the phone. Shifting from foot to foot, I fanned my face and rambled on, that it was stuffy and I needed some air.

The woman sat silently.

Continuing to chatter, I gestured toward the glass doors.

Looking down at paperwork, the woman answered, "I'll let you know."

Well, this place obviously didn't hire folks for their winning ways. I pushed open the heavy glass door and stepped into the muggy, mild air. Late January and it felt more like spring, a hint of pale sun peeping through the low lying clouds. I leaned back against the cold, concrete wall, closed my eyes and silently prayed for Mark to be all right. Our family doctor had referred Mark to the surgeon who was at the University of Florida's teaching hospital, Shands, in Gainesville, which was a bit of a drive. Mark's brother, a doctor in New England had strongly suggested we go there. He'd vetted the surgeon and declared him okay, not Boston, he reminded us, but top notch in Florida. So, even if it was something really awful, I couldn't bring myself to say the big 'C' word, he would make it; he was in good hands, young and healthy, a family who needed him and a host of reasons to live. I opened my eyes, checked my watch and went back inside asking if Mr. Hayes had come out.

Eventually, the woman glanced up, tossed her head and assured me he had not.

The stagnant pool of coffee tossed in the trash, I plopped down, stared vacantly at the faded landscapes decorating the walls and began to fidget with a frayed edge on my sweater.

"Mrs. Hayes, they're ready for you. You can go on in."

I hopped up, grabbed my bag and headed down the long, windowless corridor into the clinic area, my heels echoing a grim tattoo on the scared linoleum.

Mark was waiting, propped up on the wall outside of the open clinic room door.

One glance and I knew the news was not good. He sighed, his eyes on the space above my head.

"Mark." My hand rested on his arm, "What did the doctor say?"

"He told me to wait here. Said he'd be back in a minute. I couldn't stand to stay in the room," he added, his eyes shifting to the door. "He wanted to eyeball the fluid under the microscope."

"Well, what did he think? He must have said something."

Just then the doctor came out of a room down the hall, "Mr. Hayes, let's go in here." He nodded sideways to the room across the hall.

Two worn chairs stood sentinel in front of a metal desk.

"Have a seat."

We sat down while the doctor perched on the desk.

"Well, I wish I had better news, but it looks like a non- Hodgkin's lymphoma."

I reached for Mark's hand.

Mark's head fell to his chest. He stared at the floor.

"I know that sounds bleak, but it isn't entirely. These are usually treatable. The lump is still small and generally when they grow so rapidly, as this one has, believe it or not that's a good sign." He waited.

Neither of us spoke.

"I'll also schedule a CAT scan to make sure the cancer is contained in this one spot. I want to do the surgery quickly and remove the whole tumor, then we'll probably start an aggressive treatment of chemotherapy. Of course, we'll know more once the frozen section is back from pathology."

Stunned, I said nothing.

Mark lifted his head. "What kind of time line am I looking at? I mean, what's the prognosis with chemotherapy?"

"Fair to good. I can't be specific until I get in there and see the extent of the involvement, but from a bird's eye view with the aspirate I'd say more good than fair."

He paused, reassuring, his voice steady, "Chemo's no picnic, but it works, especially in someone young and healthy. In the 70's this would have been a death sentence, but in the last fifteen years or so we've done wonders with chemotherapy drugs."

Mark inhaled deeply then let out a long sigh, "Well, doesn't look like I have much of a choice. So let's get this over with. When can you do it?"

"I'll have the nurse book the first available."

I let go of Mark's hand and leaned forward. "Does he have to stay overnight? I mean, it's surgery and…"

"We'll get him a room just in case. It depends. You'll probably go home that evening but let's wait and see."

I opened my mouth to pose another question when the doctor bent over and laid his hand on my shoulder, promising Mark was good hands and this was serious, but the outlook encouraging. He knew we both had a lot of questions, and he'd be better able to answer them after he saw what we were dealing with. He turned to Mark, shook his hand and left the room.

Getting up I placed my arms gently around Mark's neck and my lips brushed his hair. "I don't know what to say. It'll be all right. I just know it will. Whatever happens we'll make it. In the end, I know it's going to be okay."

Motionless in the chair, Mark rested his head against my stomach, "We'll just have to wait and see."

"Hey, you have to believe it's curable, that's half the battle."

"I know, but there's a lot we don't know yet."

"There is, but the doctor said the prognosis is good. We're both in shock, and scared, but we have to believe that you will be all right."

"Just give it a rest," he paused, "please." He stood up and jerked open the door, the words ushering him out, "I've been told that I've got cancer, and you're telling me it's going to be okay. Sometimes your Pollyanna bullshit is too much."

Hot tears stung my eyes, while I watched as he was swallowed up by the mouth of the ominous hall. Silently, I followed and stopped at reception, offering the excuse of him not feeling well, and told them we'd call later to set up the surgery.

Mark sat in the car on the passenger side, his head resting on the neck brace. Looking straight ahead, he handed me the keys.

He fingered the bandage on his neck. "It's starting to hurt where they put the needle in." He managed a weak smile, "Look, I'm sorry I blew up in there. I don't need to take it out on you. Do you mind driving?"

"Oh, Mark." I leaned over, eyes overflowing and put both hands on his face pulling him in. I brushed his cheek with my lips. "I'm sorry. It's okay, it's really okay. I'm scared too." I paused, "Did he give you anything for pain?"

"No. I'll take something when we get home."

"It'll be almost two hours before we get home. Why don't I get something from the nurse? It'll just take a minute."

"No, I want to go home."

Later that evening when the children and Mark were in bed, I sat on the porch and nursed a glass of red wine. The fan above worried the still, dank air. I could smell the rain moving in, wet, heavy and pungent, reminding me of the day I first met Mark.

Like a fickle lover, spring flirted with Martha's Vineyard, the sun winking between wooly grey clouds, the air expectant with the promise of rain. Skies hovered over the choppy water at Menemsha Bite; overcast, thick, sticky and close, ozone strong in the air, the village of Menemsha, New England quaint, carefully drawn in shades of grey, blending with the sky.

I coasted down the winding hill, my bike clattering on the uneven boards of the battered dock which jutted out into the shadowy water, the outline of Cuttyhunk Island faint in the distance.

Beads of sweat dripped in my eyes, burning, the sun warm on my exposed lily white, winter skin. A native Floridian, I would never get used to the sight of my anemic looking limbs as they emerged like new hatchlings from the nest of coverings necessary for survival in the Boston winters.

Standing on the weathered dock, the rain trickled and I gratefully lifted my sweaty face up to the cooling drizzle. Whoever coined that term, 'glistening' to describe southern women when they perspired? I sweated with the best of them. Without warning the clouds opened up to a pelting downpour. Moving fast, I shoved my bike under an awning. Soaked, my tee shirt clung to my chest, and rivulets of water rushed down my face as I hunkered, drenched. I was staying at the hostel in West Tisbury and had a good ride ahead of me. When the rain finally let up, I set off, chilled but determined. Finally, I reached the hostel only to find that in my short absence it had been overrun with screeching high schoolers. Tired, wet and cranky, I was in no mood to be surrounded by inner city Boston teens. I worked in a teen center in Charlestown and had come to the Vineyard for a break, before starting grad school in the upcoming summer term.

Working for a Zen moment, I decided to just ignore them when my roommate, a fellow single woman traveler stormed in the hallway. "Someone used my hair dryer! Got it off the bunkbed and just used it like it was theirs!" She yelled up the stairs, "Hey! Chaperone or whoever is with this crowd, I need to talk to you. Now!"

A tall, ruggedly handsome man came briskly down the stairs. In a voice heavy with New England, he smiled, his deep blue eyes crinkling. "Hi, I'm Mark Hayes, the guy who brought this on. What did they do now?"

"Someone took my hair dryer off my bed, used it and left it in the bathroom. That's not okay."

"It's not okay and I'm really sorry. Is it broken?"

"I don't think so, I just want them to not get into my stuff."

"Yeah, we leave our things out and trust that no one will bother them," I added, looking up at him.

Again, he apologized and then, asked our names.

"Well, Diane and Kathy, We'll be out of here all day tomorrow and tonight the guy with me is in charge. So, to make up, can I buy you a drink? I've got my truck."

Diane and I looked at each other and she declined. She was leaving early in the morning.

He turned to me. "Will you join me? We can go over to Edgartown. The Harborside is a good place to watch a storm and it looks like one is coming in." He paused and smiled, "That is, if you like storms."

Flustered, I stammered, that I liked storms.

Nervous, quiet in the cab of his beat up pick up, I was determined not to be chatty, a trait bred into southern women from infancy; pregnant pauses to be avoided at all costs. I sat still.

He finally spoke asking me the usual where I was from. My accent sort of gave me away. Trying to sound in control, I replied, Cambridge, then added that I wasn't really from there.

"Nevah would have guessed that," he good naturedly shot back, stealing a sideways glance at me.

"Well, I guess to y'all Yankees we all sound alike," I drawled, exaggerating my slight accent. "I'm from Jacksonville, north Florida."

"And you awl eat grits and love Jimmy Carter," he smiled. "You work in Boston?"

"I do. And I eat grits and love Jimmy and am starting grad school at Tufts this summer."

"Good school. Where do you work now?"

"At a teen center in Charlestown." I grinned, and raised my eyebrows with the coincidental news.

He laughed. "And you were getting away, and I brought them all here."

"Yep, "I smiled back.

"That's kinda funny."

"Haha," I teased. "Why did you bring them all here?"

"I teach high school, and this crowd couldn't afford to go on the senior trip, so in some moment of insanity, I volunteered. Inner city kids experience nature." He laughed, "I know. It's insane. I'm insane. Honestly, I felt sorry for them." He tilted his head towards me, his eyes still on the road. "I'm a bleedin heart."

"Wow, I'm impressed."

He glanced over. "Really?"

"Well, yeah. It's nice of you, thoughtful."

"It wasn't that hard. I'll be here all summer, I'm building a house over on Chappy. It'll be rental income when I'm not using it. The land was cheap before the Ted Kennedy thing."

That evening was our beginning. The courtship flourished all summer, the Vineyard days and nights magical. We dug quahogs on Chappaquiddick, picnicked at the end of Cape Pogue and made love in the field outside Mark's house. I traveled back and forth on the bus from Boston, barreling through the dark to the ferry at Wood's Hole, school and my graduate assistantship keeping me in the city.

Fall came and we were both back in town. Mark tended to be at my apartment more than he was at his, so after Christmas we moved in together; not an easy transition. He kept late hours, often not coming home until near dawn and seemed to never have any money. In early summer, I told him to leave.

I knew he had demons; he was up front about how he had slept around with both men and women, but therapy seemed to be working for him. Gone for a couple of months, he came back.

"I don't want to do this thing without you. I'm a better man with you. I'd been lost for a long time and when I'm with you, I'm not so much. I swear to you, the craziness is over. We'll both talk to my shrink if you have doubts. I want you to marry me."

That Christmas, engaged, we went south to meet my kinfolks. Like many Yankees, Mark had been to Florida, but he'd never been to the real South. In Georgia, at my aunt's house the young black man who stayed with her came to take his suitcase.

Once we were alone, Mark erupted, incredulous at the idea of an African American servant. "Good God, did Reconstruction pass this place by or what? I seem to remember something about emancipation!"

"Please stop. It's Clenard's job to do stuff around the house. He gets paid and stays here for free, and," I paused for him to take it in, "it's how he can go to the local college. I've known him my whole life and he and Big Lucy are real tight. That's hard for outside folks to understand. She and my uncle took him in when he had no place to go, and he's been here ever since."

"Well, it's uncomfortable as hell having a guy like the kids I used to teach cart my bags."

"I know, but it is what it is. It isn't going to change anything, making him uncomfortable too." I waited then went on, "In the north, racism is just less obvious. Y'all are all about equality, yet how many black folks live on the cape next to your folks?"

The wedding was in late May on the Vineyard in the garden of an old family friend, off Dyke road, by the bridge where Kennedy had gone over; me, an only child, my small Southern Baptist family with Mark's large Yankee Catholic, lace curtain Irish. Mark, the baby, had two older brothers, one a physician who lived in Rhode Island, the other, with five kids lived on the south shore. His sister, married lived in Maine, and a first cousin, like a sister, had lived with them since her parents died. His folks had sold their Boston house and were on the Cape full time.

Our friend, an Episcopal minister, married us. The doctrine of Catholicism to the Southern Baptists bordered on idol worship and even some Episcopalians were a bit suspect, they wore those stoles and such. The Catholics weren't sure we were really married, no Mass and what about children? With tremendous foresight and good Yankee sense, Mark insisted on ample quantities of champagne which leveled the gathering. Everyone, including my Baptist relatives drank. It seemed champagne was different from plain old liquor.

A few years later, I was reminded how much I loved him when he brought home seven lab puppies and their mother, rescued from the multi-lane horror of the speeding Cape traffic. He'd seen small dark specks wandering on the shoulder, then a larger black shape heading disoriented into the lanes, the pups trailing close behind. Two were hit before he could stop. He literally blocked traffic and navigated between the whizzing cars picking up the mother, then the pups, never once deterred by the obstacles.

Chapter 3

Deeply asleep, crumpled over in the hospital sleeping chair, I grappled with the repetitive dream.

No one buried the dead anymore. There were too many. Their bodies and belongings piled in heaps, the putrid smells, the fetid smoke from the pyres thick. Few survived.

Glancing overhead, I stepped quickly in and out of the black shadows cast by the vultures' wings as they circled, swooping low. I pulled the head scarf down tight against my nose and mouth to mask the stench. I hurried, stumbling over the gnarled tree roots along the steep river bed, my long, tattered skirt catching on brambles, my shoes, old and worn, the buckle loose, I tripped. The shoe sucked into the sticky mud, and I slipped down the damp bank, the skirt catching on an outstretched limb, saved me from the fall into the rushing icy water.

Gasping and grabbing for a stronghold, I stared down into the murky depths where a man's lifeless body lay iridescent in the ghostly silver, his milky sightless eyes staring up. Jerking back, I heard the tearing of the cloth before I felt the whoosh, cut free from the tenuous hold; a scream caught in my throat as the tether let go.

From somewhere a voice called my name. My eyes shot open, and my head jerked up as I ran my hand around my sweaty, stiff neck pulling at the ringlets of hair that coiled Medusa like. In the hospital bed, tubes like marionette strings, attached Mark to various medicines. He finally was asleep. I had stayed the night and fallen asleep in the chair next to the bed.

The door opened a small crack. Marsha, my good friend and president of the small college where we worked poked her head in. Her short denim skirt set off her perpetually tanned legs and her expensively cut, chestnut hair, swung forward at her chin as she leaned in the doorway. Colleagues in Boston, Marsha had wooed me down to Florida to work with her at a newly established college for students with learning differences. The opportunity brought us closer to my family and provided Mark a less hectic schedule. He'd finished a graduate degree at Harvard before the kids were born and had been working full time plus two or so nights a week, which had allowed me to teach part time and be there for the children.

From the threshold, Marsha whispered, "I called, but no one answered. Were you sleeping?"

"No, come in. I must have fallen asleep and I was dreaming," I shuddered, recalling the dream. "It was a long night in the chair. And I had that Plague nightmare dream, where I'm the only one left with the dead man." I grimaced and attempted to rearrange my tousled hair. "Mark had a hard time getting to sleep. He just drifted off a few hours ago. It's good to see you." Getting up, I gave Marsha a hug, "Thank you for coming all this way. You're out early."

"You know I don't sleep. It's probably early menopause. I prowl the aisles of Publix for Ring Dings and Twinkies and then fret about my diet." Marsha smiled, holding out a grocery bag. "Don't start. I know you won't eat them. He'll be so happy to see 'real baked goods' though. How is he?"

"In pain. It was more complicated because of the location of the tumor. They took out as much as they could. We don't know anything else yet."

"Did you get any decent sleep?"

"No, not really. I dozed, but he tossed and fretted as the drug wore off. They gave him something a while ago so he calmed down. He's been out of it."

"And how are you holding up?"

"Oh," I paused, shaking my head, tears welling, "I don't know. I'm scared. I talked to the kids last night and Lucy just wanted to talk to her Daddy. I don't know what she, we, would do without him."

Marsha took me in her arms as my eyes overflowed. "Kath, I'm so sorry. But the doctors did say it was treatable," she reassured. "It'll just be getting through the next few months of hell. I swear historians will look back on our treatment of cancer like we now do with leeches. Did they say when they'd release him?"

I moved away and jerked a tissue out of the small box on the table, "No, but it will be late today sometime. We would have gone home last night, but the surgery was longer than expected."

"I know, I called your house and your dad told me you all spent the night. Are they telling you anything more now that they've taken out the lump?"

"No, but the doctor said he'd be in today sometime."

"So you don't know any more than you did?"

"Not really, only that the surgery was not as simple as they had figured."

Reaching out, Marsha took my cold hands into her warm ones and squeezed gently, "Listen, I'm here and I'll stay for a while if you want to get something to eat or go outside. Or I can run out and get you something."

"Oh Marsh, thanks, but I'm pretty freaked out. Not hungry, just worried and tired."

"I can't imagine." She paused, glancing over at Mark. "At least the home front is taken care of. Your folks are fine and the kids are loving having your mom and dad there. I stopped by and your mom was cooking with Lucy and your dad sitting outside smoking, watching Jake tear around on his Big Wheels."

From the bed, came an audible groan as Mark jerked his hand free from the IV port. Bright blood spurted out onto the sheets.

Looking around, confused, Mark mumbled, "What's happening? Am I bleeding?"

"It's all right, you just pulled, the IV out." Dropping Marsha's hands, I hurried over to the bed and tried unsuccessfully to put the tube back into the port. The blood oozed over the linens, warm and tacky, coloring my hands, the smell metallic and earthy, like wet mud.

Marsha came back from the bathroom with a towel and began dabbing up the iron colored flow as it seeped on the sheets.

"I called the nurse. They're coming," I said, holding the IV tube.

The door to the room swung open and the nurse came in. She stared at us, said nothing and crossed the room to the bed. Quickly pulling on gloves and a mask she had in her pocket, she adjusted the IV and covered the stained sheets with a clean blanket. Mark had closed his eyes and seemed to be out again.

"Do you all call housekeeping to clean this up?" I asked the nurse, gesturing to the stained bedding and towel.

"No," she shrugged, stepping back from the bed and removing her mask. "He's leaving today, right."

"Yes, as soon as we hear from the doctor."

The nurse's eyes darted around the room and spotted the red trash can labeled biohazard. With one swift movement she jerked off her gloves and wordlessly, disappeared into the bathroom to wash her hands. The water ran for what seemed a long time before she emerged. "The doctor should be in shortly. He's on the hall," she offered, her eyes downcast. She shoved open the door and left the room.

"Well, she was lovely," Marsha muttered, making a face. "The doctor could take an hour! I'll go see if I can find housekeeping and get this stuff cleaned up. Be right back."

"Who's here? Did I hear Marsha?" Mark's voice came weakly from the bed while he shifted sluggishly.

"Yeah, it's Marsh. Don't move around and dislodge that IV again," I sat down on the edge of the bed. "Do you want some water or anything?"

"No, I just hurt," he groaned. "God what did they do to me? I feel like I've had my head cut off. "

Fretful, I leaned down and kissed Mark lightly. "No, you're not dead yet, but they did beat you up pretty badly. You've looked better."

Marsha came back in with a hand full of towels. "Apparently, housekeeping doesn't exist in this place. No one seemed to give a damn that there is blood coagulating on the floor in here. So I'll wet these and wipe it up."

"Marsh, just leave it. We'll be gone today."

"Well, all right, if you say so," she dropped the towels on the chair. "I'll leave it, but I'd complain. This place is just awful. No one wanted to help me at all. And what's with the red sign on the door?"

"What red sign?"

"It's an 'X' with caution on the door. It's on some other doors too."

"I don't know. I haven't been out of here."

"Well, they sure as hell aren't the most helpful people. They acted like I had the Plague or something!" Marsha looked over at Mark and saw that his eyes were open. "Well, it's about time you woke up to see me. I drive all this way AND bring you sustenance, Twinkies and Ring Dings and you stay asleep." She crossed over to the bed and laid her hand on his.

Managing a weak grin, Mark answered, "You know me so well. I've always been impressed with women who don't bake."

After Marsha left, the nurse came in, donned mask and gloves and removed Mark's IV. She went out without saying anything. Mark was dressing in the bathroom, while I packed up the few things that he had brought.

The nurse returned. "The doctor isn't coming in now and before you can be officially checked out, the doctors in radiology want to meet with you both."

"Not coming in? How come? And why do they want to meet with us now?" I glanced up, tired and exasperated. "I don't want to sound rude, but we know it's lymphoma. If the final pathology report isn't back what can radiology possibly tell but what we already know?"

The nurse didn't respond.

Smashing the shaving kit down into the overnight bag I yanked the zipper closed. "We know that they didn't get it all, we can't set up chemo until they know what grade cancer it is, we're exhausted, and if the surgeon isn't coming back, why can't this wait until tomorrow or the next day?"

"All that I know is what I was told," the nurse turned away and fiddled with the blinds. "Your husband will not be released until you both meet with the doctors. Radiology is downstairs in the basement. Just follow the signs and the yellow lines on the floor."

I grabbed the handles of the bag, jerked it off the bed and slammed it down on the floor. "And we're off to see the wizard."

"Excuse me."

"Nothing, I was talking to myself."

As the nurse walked out of the room, Mark came from the bathroom dressed to leave.

"You look much better," I kissed him. "I'll get a wheelchair. You wait here."

"What was that all about with the nurse?"

"Oh, more hospital crap. They will not release 'your husband' until we both meet with the doctors."

"What? How come?"

"I couldn't get anything from her. I don't get it. These people are just rude. But we've gone this far. It'll take a few minutes and maybe we'll find out something more. Let me get the wheelchair."

"No. No, I need to walk. I want to get this over with."

Mark move slowly out the door and I followed carrying the overnight satchel.

"We go to the basement and follow the yellow lines."

When we reached the elevator Mark rested against the wall, his eyes closed.

"Are you all right? I think you need a chair."

"No. I'm okay."

My eyes filled with hot, angry tears. "I hate that you have to go through this. I can't do it all alone without you. Lucy and Jake need their daddy. I need you."

"I need you all too, I always have." Bending down he kissed me and held my hand as the elevator stopped. "I hurt," he sighed, "and I'll hurt more before all of this is over. I just have to trust I'll make it, that we'll make it."

We got out and turned left following the signs for radiology. Down a long, dank institutional corridor, the yellow lines on the floor guided us to a reception desk.

"My husband and I were told to meet some doctor here from radiology. He's just had surgery and is pretty wiped out."

The woman glanced up from her papers, "Well, have a seat and I'll see what's going on. Do you know who the doctor is?"

"No, they sent us down here from upstairs and said that the hospital wouldn't release him until we met with someone from here."

Moving away from the counter I shoved the overnight bag under the chair and plopped down next to Mark.

"These people are not one bit helpful. I really don't get it. You just had surgery and no one seems to care or know anything."

"Honey, let it go. It doesn't matter. We'll be out of here in a while."

"You're right. Nothing actually matters but you getting better."

"We're both wiped out. Don't spend any energy on being angry. It won't help."

We sat quietly for a few minutes and a nurse came out. Looking around the waiting room, her eyes fixed on me and Mark, "Mr. and Mrs. Hayes."

Mark slowly got up, standing still for a moment to steady himself. I moved to help him but he shook his head, "I'm all right."

We followed the nurse down a short narrow hall into a large windowless room. The hospital green walls surrounded a cold steel examining table and overhead a bright fluorescent light buzzed, the bulb ready to go. To the right of the table sat a metal stool and a battered desk. Beside the desk, a lone padded chair, the armrests fraying. Holding carefully to the arms, Mark eased down in the chair.

I stood by the long table. "What an awful room." My eyes shot up and rested on the humming light. "It's like the Milgram experiment without the white coats. It's creepy and cold and that buzzing sound is terrible. Whom do you suppose we're seeing?"

Abruptly, the door opened and two women and a man wearing white coats came into the room.

"Hello," the petite, dark haired woman leading the group nodded to Mark.

Moving away from the table, I towered over her.

"I'm Dr. Blake from radiology and this is Dr. Rosen. Dr. Davis is from oncology." She gestured first to the woman and then the man beside her.

I nodded to the doctors and as a group, they spread over to where Mark sat. Dr. Blake looked down at Mark, "Mr. Hayes, how are you?"

"You'll excuse me if I don't get up. You probably know better than I do how I feel."

"Are you feeling any better now that the anesthesia's worn off?"

"Not really, I sort of liked the drugs," he shrugged, a weak smile teasing at the corner of his mouth.

No one in the group smiled.

Dr. Blake continued, "The soreness is going to last a few days. The incision was bigger than the surgeon anticipated." She sat on the metal stool by the desk while the other two doctors remained standing.

I leaned against the wall beside Mark's chair. The only noise in the room was the buzzing from the light. No one spoke.

"Do you have more information for me? I was planning to go home."

"The biopsy came back from pathology. The frozen section will take a few days, but what we have is fairly clear, it confirms the needle aspirate. It's a non-Hodgkin's lymphoma."

"I think we knew that before," said Mark, his tone puzzled.

"Yes, well," Dr. Blake paused, staring over at him, "you realize that the surgeon couldn't get all of the tumor because of the nerves in your neck and the way the tumor was growing. It was more complicated than it showed on the CAT scan."

"I figured that."

"Chemo and radiation will be the course of treatment."

"And I will be coordinating the chemo protocol with Dr. Rosen," Dr. Davis added, nodding his head to the woman beside him, "who is in charge of the radiation treatment. We want to begin the chemo as soon as possible."

"Is the chemo IV?" I asked from my spot at the wall.

"IV and oral. We'll go over the details when you come in. I'd like to see you tomorrow," Dr. Blake responded.

"Tomorrow? But he's still hurting from the surgery."

"I know, but we need to get this started right away."

"I'll be here tomorrow," Mark injected. "I want to get this over with and the sooner I start the sooner it's done."

"I'll have the nurse put you in for late morning." Dr. Blake looked quickly at the other doctors before going on, then directly at Mark. "You and your wife need to know a piece of information that has come up as a direct result of the biopsy."

My posture shifted from weary leaning to attention, and I stepped away from the wall. The other two doctors glanced uncomfortably at Dr. Blake.

"What new information?" Mark asked.

"You are HIV positive."

Mark gaped at the woman.

Not sure of what I heard, I crossed over to Mark and rested my hand on his shoulder. "Did you just say he was HIV positive?"

The doctor nodded, "Yes."

"Well," I said, relief evident in my voice, "you have the wrong person. That's someone else's test," I clarified without doubt.

Mark's hands began to tremble. He didn't respond but fell forward in the chair and cupped his hands over his ears, shaking his head back and forth. He stopped, looked up, his voice faltering, "This doesn't make any sense."

"Mr. Hayes, do you have any idea why you might be HIV positive?" Dr. Blake asked, her eyes fixed on me.

"No," Mark hesitated, his voice trembling, "I don't know why I might be HIV positive. I've never had a blood transfusion. I'm not a drug addict."

"And we've been married for years," I shot a nasty glare at the teeny woman. "This is crazy. You all have made a horrible mistake."

"I'm sorry, but it is the correct test," the doctor responded evenly. "We rarely make mistakes like that here."

"Well, you've made one big one. It must be a false positive," I interrupted, angry now.

"Unfortunately, no. The test is never a false positive. A false negative, but not a false positive."

The incessant hum of the florescent light grew louder and the green walls started to spin. *The red sign on the doors. Now it made sense.* I clutched the corner of the metal table, closed my eyes and took in a deep breath. A bit steadier, my eyes opened, I asked, "There must be another test? I mean how accurate is this thing?"

"It's fairly accurate. There is another test, the Western Blot that we'll run of course, just to be absolutely certain, but I don't think it'll show a different result."

The bile clotted in my throat. I shook my head trying to dislodge the information I'd just been given.

Mark sat silently, staring up at the flickering overhead light.

"Well, what does this mean? Does this mean he has AIDS?" My eyes darted frantically to each doctor.

"We believe that the cancer is a result of the HIV infection."

"Does my husband have AIDS?" My voice now high pitched and frantic.

"No. Not at this point."

"But, he'll get AIDS? That's what HIV means." I was having trouble breathing. My throat was clogged, my eyes burning. Gazing down at Mark, my voice came from somewhere far away, like I was watching a movie scene unfold, and I'd belatedly, finally figured out the plot. "Does this mean I am HIV positive too?"

The doctors stood silent.

My eyes darted frantically around the room.

Dr. Blake finally spoke. "It's likely."

Mark grabbed at his bandaged neck and turned his head to face her. His voice cracked, panicked, "What about our children?"

"How old are they?"

"Five and three," he stammered.

"We don't know a lot about the disease in children, but the older they are, the less likely they're infected."

"What do you mean?" I croaked out.

"Well, chances are the five year old is fine, but the younger one may not be."

"Oh, dear God."

A locomotive barreled through my head. Blood throbbed in my ears so loudly that I clutched my hands around my neck to quiet the racing pulse. I lunged for the door, staggered out of the room into the desolate hall, crashed against the cold pocked wall and hunched over, strands of hair falling in my face, sticking to my lips. Crouching forward, I threw up.

"Mrs. Hayes." From somewhere overhead I heard my name as a white blur floated fuzzily in front of me and my eyes attempted to focus. I'd slumped down against the wall in the corridor outside the examining room, loose hair streaked with vomit dangled around my face and fetid dribbles continued down the front of my shirt. I crawled out of my safe, dark place, and wrinkled my nose at the foul odor, then realized the smell was coming from me.

Dr. Rosen reached out her hand and wearily, I got up. The doctor guided me into the bathroom. "You'll probably want to wash up," she offered and turned on the faucet, staring into my vacant image in the mirror. "I'm going to get you some water to rinse out your mouth. I'll be back in a minute."

Alone, I peered in the smudged mirror over the sink and hung there, listless, the sound of the water rushing out of the tap, like the whooshing in the Plague dream when my hold came loose. Now I had slipped into the icy grave.

This can't be happening. In a minute, I'll wake up.

The bathroom door opened and the doctor returned with a paper cup filled with water. "Rinse your mouth out and then swallow this." She opened her hand to give me a small white pill.

"What is it?"

"It's a mild sedative, Xanax. It'll help."

"Thank you, but I don't want it." I turned back to the sink and splashed water on my face. "Just leave the cup of water. Please." My back to the doctor, I pulled a paper towel from the dispenser and dampened it, swiping the stiffening reeds of hair and dabbing at the spots on my shirt.

Dr. Rosen waited, not making eye contact, glancing at the wall over my head, "I'll give you a few of the Xanax to keep, just in case. They might help." She hesitated, her brown eyes moving to me, "Is there anything that I can do for you?"

I regarded the concerned woman's reflection in the mirror. Wordlessly, I shook my head.

"Well then, I'll leave you. Your husband is outside. I'll see you in the morning to discuss the treatment."

Without turning around I responded to the woman in the mirror, "There is no treatment for this." I pushed away from the sink, brushed past the doctor and shoved open the door.

Mark waited, curled over in the chair in the reception area, his overnight bag collapsed in a heap by his feet. When he saw me he hoisted himself up, moving like an old man, his neck bandaged, his brilliant eyes, red rimmed and filled with pain. I bent down and took his bag. Walking out of the hospital, neither of us spoke.

At the car, I opened the door to the driver's side. "I'm not driving home now. I can't face my folks, and we have to be back here in the morning."

"That's fine."

We drove in silence while I pulled into a motel close to the hospital.

Once in the room, Mark lay down wearily on top of the made up bed, his hand over his eyes.

"I need to call my folks."

Mark said nothing.

On the phone by the bed, I punched in the familiar number and after a couple of rings my mother answered.

"Hi, Mom. No, yes, yes, we're all right."

My mental image was of my mother as I always thought of her. At the house I grew up in, in the kitchen, talking into the old wall phone, a vestige from the 1960s, her wavy reddish hair, graying, cut short, wisps curling around her ears.

"No, I'm just tired. He's okay, Mom. Sore and weary so we're staying here tonight. Yes, in the morning we have to meet with the other doctors. No," I hesitated, "they know it's lymphoma, and he'll start chemo right away. Sure, here he is."

"She wants to talk to you." Handing the phone to Mark I walked into the bathroom to shed my stinking clothing.

"No, I'm all right." he sighed, "Yes, tired and a bit sore, and it's not good news. Yeah, we knew it, but I always hoped. So, how are the kids? Great. No, we'll be home tomorrow. Tell them we love them. You too. Thank you. Bye"

I'd slipped on a clean T-shirt and was in bed under the covers with my eyes shut when Mark hung up the phone. He got up and crossed over to sit on the edge of the bed next to me. He gently touched my damp hair.

"This can't be real," I said to him softly, shaking my head, tears pooling in my eyes.

"I know. I talked some more to the doctors when you were outside. They'll do another test in the morning. Something called a Western Blot. It's the most accurate and the best test they have."

My voice rose, grasping onto any smidgen of hope, "Is there a chance the other test could be wrong?"

"They don't think so, but they'll run this just in case."

I rolled over on my side to face him. "It doesn't make any sense at all. How could you get AIDS?"

He dropped his head, "I don't know." He moved away from the bed and walked to face the window. "I've never really understood about prayer."

I gazed at his broad shoulders, the bandage on his neck, a fresh white cravat. I got up and crossed over to him, putting my arm around his waist and rested my head on his shoulder, "I pray."

"I know you do. And you believe."

"Yes, I believe."

"I never have."

"I know."

"Does it help?"

"It always has, but I don't know now. It can't hurt."

He turned around and looked down at me. Gently, brushing his lips on my forehead, he walked away from the window, went into the bathroom and closed the door.

Hours later, in the bed I listened to Mark's steady breathing. He had taken pain pills and was in a drugged slumber. I glanced over at the lighted clock by the bed. It was 2:00 am, and I hadn't slept at all. Getting up, I rummaged in my purse and found the medicine the doctor had given me. I went into the bathroom, filled a glass with water and swallowed one small white pill. Lying back down the drug took effect quickly and I floated above the bed.

Maybe this is like dying, I thought and closed my eyes.

Chapter 4

The chemical poisoning had stopped and the chemo driven, violent, vomiting surges finally ended. We had a respite from the long, excruciating trips to the hospital and a short reprieve before the radiation treatments began. Thankfully, there was a radiation oncologist nearby whom the hospital recommended, so as debilitating as the radiation would no doubt be, at least we would be home.

Gaunt, Mark's skin was a translucent grey and his remaining hair stuck out in odd angles like one of those shriveled apple dolls that sell at fall festivals.

I wandered through the motions of living in a thick Xanax haze of half-truths and constant dread. This was 1989, central Florida, where earlier, a family further south had been thrown out of their school district and had their house burned because their two boys, both hemophiliacs had AIDS. Fear of the virus and lack of knowledge about how it was contracted were very real.

Scared to share the real story with anyone, including family, only the necessary few knew the truth. Mark's brother helped negotiate the medical maze; Marsha, covered for me at work, and Mike, a pediatrician friend in Boston, remained on alert for signs of the illness in the children.

The small college community, sympathetic to the horrible news of Mark's cancer rallied around our family. Sam, a young faculty colleague took my classes, students volunteered to babysit, and my childhood friend, Annie and her little boy came frequently to be with the kids. Neighbors brought dinners, and both of our families called almost daily. Fraught with worry that someone would find out the truth, I dodged questions and avoided well- meaning overtures.

Days began heralded with new doubts. If Lucy or Jake had a cold or tummy ache, I figured it was the beginning of the illness. Assurance from the local pediatrician, who didn't have the true story, and Mike, up north, that the children were healthy, did little. The only way to allay the fears was for me to get tested and that was not even certain. For the test to be accurate, you had to wait for about nine months from the time of infection, which was an unknown. I constantly scrutinized spots on my skin, panicked if I had diarrhea and checked my mouth for fungal infections three or four times a day if my throat happened to be scratchy.

Little in life mattered to me. My world now consisted of struggling through each day. I rallied for birthdays, Lucy turned six and Jake four. I cooked, but ate little and swallowed Xanax with a wine chaser nightly. Jake would run to me excited about some new discovery only to retreat dejected when I shrugged a weak 'that's nice, sweetie.' I knew that the children needed time and attention, and that I should break up with my new best friend, Xanax ... soon.

School finished for the children and Boston friends offered their condo in Boca Grande. The island held pleasant memories for us and was an easy drive.

It was also close enough that my parents could visit us there for a couple of days. I had insisted they visit infrequently during the chemo, my excuses, flimsy; the house was small, Mark was up all night, horribly sick, I'd need them later, whatever reason I could come up with, and they had acquiesced. I couldn't tell them until I knew what I was facing and had put them off during most of the chemo. Couching the truth in half lies had been hell over the past months. Face to face, it would be even harder to keep the truth from them.

The shock on my parents' faces when they saw Mark was palpable. Even my mother's southern charm was inadequate at masking her disbelief when she first saw him. My dad was direct and caring. He asked Mark lots of questions, and then talked about the weather and fishing. I noticed that he made the gin and tonics much stronger that evening.

While the men chatted, Mom took me aside in the kitchen. Standing over the sink, her hands sticky with crabmeat she said gently, "I know this is awful for you, and all of us, but you need to pull yourself together. You're not eating, not sleeping and have even stopped talking. Mark is a strong, young man who can beat this." She turned to me, "Honey, you're acting like you're the one with cancer. You have to be there for Mark and the kids."

I leaned on the counter, avoiding her scrutiny.

"I know you're scared and with good reason. The idea of raising two children alone and losing the man you love is terrible, but you're brave and healthy and whatever happens you can cope with it." Wiping her hands on the towel, she reached out and put her arms around me, "You just have to have faith."

I can't tell her the truth, she can't take it. If I get sick then she'll have to know, but I can't tell her this way. I smiled weakly and returned her hug, "I know. I'm okay, just tired and the past months have been so hard. It's good to have you and Daddy here." My eyes filling, I fled the kitchen.

My dad, his long frame draped over the club chair in the next room was smoking his pipe, feet propped up on the ottoman, the sound of the water coming in through the open porch door. Retired from his full time job as an editor, he still worked a couple of days a week and had settled into a routine that gave him time for gardening, puttering and a bit of travel with my mom.

"Hey, darling," he smiled, his steel grey eyes crinkled into the well-drawn crow's feet when he saw me coming into the room. "I opened the door to hear the waves and," he winked, nodding his head in the direction of the kitchen door, "she won't fuss so much about the smell. If it gets too hot in here we'll close the door and I'll put the pipe out." He paused. "I should have lived near the water. Never get tired of the sound." He took a draw on his pipe. "Mark and the kids are out in the pool. Come sit down," he patted the footstool.

I sat as he adjusted his feet and put his pipe on the side table. Inhaling his scent, old cherries and clean clothes, I catapulted back to childhood. My dad had been my constant, my north star. Whenever I was afraid, he was always there, promising me that I'd find my way home. My throat tightened, eyes stung and the tears welled up.

One look and Dad reached out, taking me in his arms. I fell to my knees beside the chair, my head on his knee, weeping softly while he held me and stroked my hair with his large, rough hand. He didn't speak, just moved his hand rhythmically back and forth like he had done when I was little and had gone to him with my tears.

"There, there."

I looked at him through the mist of water gathering on my lashes.

"It'll be all right."

For a moment, I felt the power of my father's belief and a fleeting peace settled. I held his gaze, time suspended, over in seconds. "Oh, Daddy, I hope so," I breathed.

"Mommy! Guess what we did!" The moment gone. Mark and children had returned from the pool, Teenage Mutant Ninja Turtles blasted on TV, and the perceived normalcy of Mom's crab cakes and bed.

The time on the island didn't provide the hoped for reprieve. After my parents left, Lucy and I got sick with an incapacitating stomach bug. The trip off island to the doctor was a trek and afraid of what I might find out, decided to tough it out.

Jake, the only one of us unaffected by illness, jumped in and out of the pool and chased the seagulls up and down the beach.

Depleted by the latest round of chemotherapy, Mark floated in the pool wearing a large sun hat to protect his bare head and slept on and off in fitful little naps. Jake's boundless energy only seemed to irritate him.

When Jake started crying about why was Daddy so grouchy, I dragged myself out of bed. My suspicion was that this was the beginning of the virus, but I tried to keep up a brave front for the children. Wiping Lucy's face after another bout of her throwing up, I couldn't quell the tears.

Concerned, her child voice insistent, Lucy asked, "When is Daddy going to be better? I hate it when he is sick. I want things to be like they were before." She stretched out her chubby arms and threw them around my neck, "You're always sad now, Mommy."

I clung protectively to her small body, "Oh sweetie, I'll try not to be so sad. Daddy will be better," I assured her, trying to believe my own words.

The next day, the vomiting and diarrhea had stopped, but I couldn't shake the fear that the virus was rearing its head.

Thankfully, Lucy was back to normal. She ate a huge supper and pronounced, "Now that we're all better it's time for ice cream".

"Pleeeease," Jake jumped down from his chair, hopped in Mark's lap, begging, "Daddy, can we pleease, pleease go to the Pink Pony?"

"Okay, guys, calm down." Mark grinned, "I'll take you if you promise not to argue about who gets shotgun."

I didn't feel up to going and sat on the porch, contemplating the remaining Xanax, overlooking the water, while the sun began its show stopping descent.

When they got back, Mark saw me still sitting there and started the children's baths and tucked them in bed, telling them I'd be along in a few minutes. Carrying two drinks, a gin and tonic for me, and his usual, Jameson's, straight up, he plopped down in the chair across the table from me and handed me the drink with a wry smile, "As Annie would say, it's a stump lifter."

Taking a sip I raised my eyebrows, "You hit me mighty hard. You know what a lightweight I am." I took another sip peering at him from under my eyelids, "A cheap drunk, I believe were your words."

"That's only when you threw up in the car." Shaking his head, he laughed, "I actually married the woman who threw up in my new car and danced on tables at MY high school reunion."

I took another swig. "This is strong," I looked out at the water, "but it will do the trick. I figure if I drink enough it will make me forget for a while. And then, when I take my magic pill I'll go to a happier place."

"Kathy, don't."

I glanced over at Mark. "I'm sorry. I am such a baby. You are sick, dying and here I am whining."

He leaned across the table and took my hand. "I can't stand to see you like this. You've checked your mouth at least five times today. You don't eat or sleep. You're making yourself crazy. And you will get sick. Not from AIDS but from worry and exhaustion."

Letting go of his hand, I stared down into my drink and stirred it silently with my index finger. Not looking up I answered Mark softly, "I feel so horrible. I watch you each day and don't know how you cope. You've been through so much already and it's just begun." I lifted my eyes to him.

He shook his head.

In a rush of words, I continued, "I'm like the whiny, spoiled child you accuse me of being when we argue."

"No," he paused, "no, you're not."

"But I am." I bent forward, elbows on the table, "I think about myself and get mad at you that you're sick. You didn't choose to get sick. You have no idea how or when you got this and now you're the one who is sick, yet you don't complain, you just suck it up and go on."

"No, I'm not that heroic. I go on because I don't know what else to do."

"You know," I fell back in the chair and gazed at the water, "we probably all have it. You got it so long ago that I'd have to be infected and if I have it the kids do too. The doctors' weren't real hopeful, especially about Jake."

"No, I don't think they have it. The kids are healthy."

"For now and now doesn't matter for long, so I just wait and try to pray, which hasn't been that easy lately, because there's nothing anyone can really do, is there?" I ran my hand down the sweating glass, "All the drugs they have just make you sick and maybe buy a few months."

My voice broke. I stumbled on, "Every time the kids or I get anything, I think it's the beginning of the disease. No one understands why I'm so panicked. People at work just stare at me and think, *oh poor thing, her husband has cancer and she just can't cope.*"

Mark said nothing.

"The other day one of the secretaries said in this sugary, over concerned voice, *'It must be nice to be so close to your husband. You seem so worried and preoccupied all of the time it's like you have cancer too.'* I glared at her and mumbled something like yes, we are very close. "The truth is I really can't cope."

"But you are coping. It doesn't matter what people think."

"No, I'm not," I shook my head. "I'm terrified all of the time. Hardly a moment passes that I don't remember we may not be all right. I've had this recurring dream. In the dream, it's way back in time, but this feels like, it's like in the dream," I hesitated, "I'm hanging on a ledge and below is a freezing rushing river. The bank is giving way. I'm slipping off the ledge and the ground crumbles underneath me. I can't stop it." Closing my eyes I took a deep breath, not telling him about the rest of the dream with the dead man in the river, "And it hurts so bad on the way down."

"Don't do this," Mark reached across the table both hands extended palms up.

I opened my eyes, resting my hands in his upturned palms. "No, I want to say this." My voice rose as I went on, intent, "You know at this point the idea of dead is meaningless. By the time this is all over, death will be welcome. It's the pain that will come before it that I can't imagine." I shook my head, "You know what a baby I am. I just think about what you've gone through already, and then think, my God, it's nothing compared to what you, we could face. I look at the kids and I can't even see them. I'm petrified, Mark." My throat clogged, the familiar hot tears welled up. "Not just scared, like it will be over soon, but really terrified."

I lurched out of the chair and crossed the porch arms hugging my body, my back to Mark. "I don't have the gumption or faith or whatever it is to watch them suffer and not be able to do anything." I faltered, "I think, I really think I would do something. Something awful, something like kill myself and the kids before I would watch them die a horrible death."

"Don't say that." The words echoed from the shadowy corner.

I whirled around to face him, my back against the fine mesh screen, "Why not? I know that I could. I would kill to save my children. Maybe, even to save them pain. And I would, I think I really would." I inhaled, weighing my words, "It frightens me to know that. But I know that."

Turning away, I stared out at the water. It was indigo now. What was left of the blazing sun had cast its color wash over the horizon and the evening sky's ultraviolet haze hovered over the darkening water. I came back to the table and reached for the dripping glass, tears burning my eyes.

Mark's quiet voice broke the silence, "I know you don't want to get tested yet and don't want to know if you have it, but what if you don't have it. If you don't, then the kids don't, and you can be free of this. I can understand you not wanting to know, but you may not have it."

"It won't be a valid test, not now, it's too soon. Remember, I asked Dr. Davis all about it." I sipped my drink. "We didn't have sex a lot after Jake, but I know we did a few times last fall before the lump showed up. We used a condom but that's not foolproof. You were diagnosed in late January. It's only the end of June. To be really accurate, not get a false negative, you have to wait for about a year." I swallowed, trying to keep the tears back. "Anyway, what good would it all do?" Watching him in the grey blue light, my voice faltered. "I don't want to know that we're going to die."

Crying, I buried my head in my arms on the table. Mark got up and came around the table, and tenderly touched my arm. *His hands are cold. Cold and dry like an abandoned shell. He's always cold now. Even his touch is gone. And the disease has only begun. Oh God, please help me. He's trying so hard to help me and it's happening to him.* Tears running down my cheeks, I lifted my head and covered his cold hand with my warm one.

"I'll get tested in the fall and we'll go from there." *I'll try not to look in my mouth so much. I'm so selfish and pitiful. I know it must be awful for you when you are feeling so lousy to see me worry so.* "I'll try to be better. I promise."

"You don't need to try to be better, I'm just worried about you. It's just that, well, I wish you'd get tested because I think you're okay. I think the kids are too. The only way they can be infected is through you, at birth and I really believe that you're not sick."

"Dearest, Mark," I shot him a weak smile and grasped his hand, "you want us to be all right so badly. But you got this probably years ago. It's not likely that I haven't picked it up at some point." I managed a weak smile. "Our sex life was pretty hot, remember? You have no other risk factors even though you did sleep around in your 20's, as did many people. It was the seventies, after all. We've gone through this so many times. You or the doctors can't pinpoint anything."

"Kathy, listen to me." Mark held my eyes with his voice. "I can't stand to see you like this. I love you. I've loved you from that first time at the hostel when you were dripping wet and mad." He gently tucked a stray hair behind my ear. "Anyway, you can't go on not sleeping, not eating, living on Xanax and panicked all of the time."

He dragged his chair over. "There's something I need to tell you. I'm taking a huge risk here, but I'm counting on what we have to get us through this. You might, well, never mind that, anyway, I think that you and the kids are okay," he put his hand on my knee, "because I might know when I may have gotten this."

Speechless, I stared at him.

"So... you remember after Jake was born I used a rubber. You hated it, but I said I didn't want another kid. Well, that was true. And..." He removed his hand and looked away. "It's that well, I've tried. I've fought it, but it didn't do any good. I found myself going for the rush, the incredible rush I've always gotten with sex, with men and with women, but more so, with men. It's not about love, it's not intimate, it's a hot, fast come. It's why our sex life has sucked for so long."

Dumbfounded, I opened my mouth to speak.

"No, don't say anything. I've got to do this. If I stop now, I'll never finish what I need to say." He continued, still not looking at me. "You knew that I'd been with men before, and I've never had a relationship with any of them. I'm not gay. It's only sex, and it never really affected us. You were enough for a while, more than anyone ever had been. With you it was love, passion, but somehow not the same rush that I got with men." He paused to take a breath.

Not trusting what I'd just heard, I rapidly injected, "Wait. Let me get this right." Each word controlled, my voice trembled, "You think that you got AIDS from a man, after Jake was born." My hand crept to my mouth muffling the next words. "And Jake and Lucy may be okay, because I probably didn't have it when they were born."

Mark nodded.

"And you think, I don't have it now, because the times that we had sex before you got sick, those times, you used a condom, because you thought about it, you wondered. Is that what you're telling me?" In disbelief, I stared at him.

He nodded, "Yes, that's what I'm telling you. It's why I think you and the kids are okay. We've probably only had sex a few times since Jake was born. Remember we were always tired with the two of them, and then I had that ulcer thing."

"Did you have ulcers or was that AIDS?"

"I don't know."

"Do the doctors know any of this?"

"No, no one knows."

"Who was he?" I shot the question into the murky darkness.

"I don't know. It was just sex. We didn't exchange names."

The water slapped rhythmically at the dock. It was the only sound, the usual symphony of night noises, silent. In the distance, the boat lights across the harbor blinked on and off and a warm breeze danced over the tops of the mangroves.

I sat stunned, listening to the uncanny night quiet.

Mark remained motionless in his chair staring at nothing.

When I spoke again, my words came out slow and deliberate. "You know, it makes more sense now, you not wanting me." Like a blinding flash, I thought about his always being tired, the late work nights, the phone calls with the hang ups, seeing a car like his at a rest area and his denial that it wasn't his car.

Mark's handsome, shadowy features were outlined in the glimmering moonlight as he replied, "No. It wasn't like that. I wanted you, but I couldn't stop wanting others too. No one person was ever enough."

I knocked back what was left of my drink deliberately setting down the glass. "You know, you never drink too much. I always envied you that. You were so in control, so not like me." Stopping, I looked out at the shimmering water then back at him. "But then, there's always been that other part of you, hasn't there? The part that I never understood. That I wasn't privy to, the moodiness." I paused. "I wonder if you even knew what it was. But that's silly isn't it? Of course you knew, you just fought it and kept it down for a while."

I got up from the table and began to pace back and forth in front of the screen. "Tell me." I spun around facing him. "I believe that I have a right to know, I think. How long had we been married when this started?"

Mark peered off in the black distance, "About two years."

I stopped moving. "My God, this has been going on for almost eight years? After all the therapy bullshit! I really am stupid."

"No, it's really not like that," he pleaded. "It's hard to explain. I love you. I've never, not loved you. It's like," he stammered, "it's like I'm an addict and I can't help it. No one is ever enough, not you, not any of them. No one." His eyes filled with tears. "I hoped you could understand. This has been hell. You don't know what it's been like for me. And I'm going to die."

I had retreated to the end of the porch. Mark's silent profile magnified against the dimly lit backdrop of the porch, the tears coursing down his cheeks, his shoulders shuddering as he cried.

I studied him, unable to say anything. Finally, from the dark distance I asked, "So you knew? You knew when the cancer diagnosis came that it wasn't just cancer?"

"No. I wasn't sure. I was scared."

"But you knew in the doctor's office. You knew how you got it."

"I didn't really know."

"But you knew you had been screwing around. You could have gotten infected anytime in all those years!"

"I told you, I couldn't help it."

I exploded, "You couldn't help it? Oh my God! You played Russian Roulette with our lives and you couldn't fucking help it?"

"No! It wasn't like that. I never meant to hurt you or the kids. It was just sex. I love you. I never thought this would happen. I didn't want to die!"

"Why didn't you just leave me? Men realize they're gay all the time."

"That's not it. I'm not gay."

I raged on, "Or even, God forgive me, even kill yourself if you were so tormented that you couldn't help yourself." *You could have made it look like an accident. You know it would better than this. You would have been mourned.*

"Please, don't do this," he pleaded.

I sheltered in the protective recesses of the porch, my voice catching, my hand brushing back the wisps of hair catching in my mouth. "Of course, we would have been stunned. Everyone shocked. But then," I inhaled and rushed on, "as time passed you would have been remembered as a good man, a brilliant scholar cut down before his time, tortured by unknown demons, a wonderful father, a loving husband."

I stopped and turned away from him, looking out at the night. "I would have been devastated and wondered where I'd screwed up, but then, then it would have been over. I would have gone on, different, missing you, not untarnished. But not like this, like we are now- some unknown malignancy, festering, waiting, spreading and in the end devouring us."

Mark stood up and walked over to the shadows where I was still, my rant finished.

I whirled around.

"Kathy, don't do this, don't do this to us. Please. I knew telling you was a risk, but I couldn't bear to watch you like you were. I love you."

Hovering motionless, I was lost in a space somewhere past him.

He put his arms around me. "You said in the hospital we would weather this and we can. We have to for the kids." He tilted my chin, my face to his, "I know that I've hurt you. I've hurt all of us. All I want to do is to live long enough to make it up to you and to the kids. Don't let your anger take you away from me, please. I need you."

He rested his head on my shoulder, and the wetness from his tears dampened my shirt.

As we stood, his arms around me, I absently stroked his head where the downy new growth of hair was coming in. *It's coming in so dark.*

Completely void of any feeling that I could identify, I left my body and viewed myself from afar. Strange, it brought some relief, distance from the horror coupled with a searing, burning pain and then emptiness.

Mark's voice came from somewhere out there. "I'm tired. I've got to go to bed. Come soon, please."

Vaguely aware that he'd left, I went into the kitchen, poured straight gin over ice, took it back to the porch and watched the water, seeing nothing until the sun that I had seen go down, come up, and cast its purplish, gray net over the damp dawn.

Wandering sleepily out onto the porch, Jake climbed on my lap and kissed me on the cheek. He smelled warm and damp, fresh from his dreams, his hair moist around his temples. I gazed down at the bronzed, tow headed little boy clad in his new favorite Ninja Turtle Pajamas.

"Did you see any dolphins yet, Mommy?"

Not speaking, I grasped him tightly, my heart aching with love.

"Mommy, you're hurting me. Where's Daddy." He wriggled away and ran into the house. Slowly, I got up, stiff from the hours sitting in the chair and followed him.

Chapter 5

Back at home I tenuously balanced the tasks of living with a new truth. Knowing that the children were probably safe lessened my worry, but the reality that I could be infected was never far from my mind. The outrage and disbelief over what had been going on all these years threatened to consume me. In addition to the immense betrayal, I wondered how could I have been so stupid, so blind? And then, like a sympathetic anti-hero, there was Mark, frightened, miserable and suffering, the father of my children, the man I had loved.

Feebly, trying to balance work, kids and this insane life, I carted Mark back and forth to the nightmare of daily radiation treatments and watched helplessly as the deadly rays scorched his throat. The one blessing was that I only had to drive a few miles. We were finished with the mega hospital that was Shands.

Seeing Mark in such bad shape after a couple of weeks, I told the local radiologic oncologist, Dr. Jacobsen that I wasn't sure how much more of this my husband could tolerate.

He acknowledged that while the protocol was tough, Mark was holding up fairly well, particularly with his immune system so depleted.

What little energy Mark had gained back after the chemo had come to an abrupt halt with the new treatment. Angry burn marks appeared on his throat and his lips were constantly parched from the close proximity of the blistering light. Direct hits from the radiation affected his vocal cords and his voice grew weak and raspy. He slept most of the time.

I finally broke down, tearing up, when Dr. Jacobsen came into the room. He pulled out a chair and got a box of tissues off the desk. "Let's chat a minute." He sat beside me on a small stool. "I know how Mark is doing, but I'm concerned about you. How're you holding up?"

I managed a weak, "I'm not. Holding up that is. I barely get through the day. And I see Mark losing more every day, and I think I'm going to get sick soon and the kids…"

"For what it's worth, your kids are most likely fine. They're older and healthy. We don't know that much about this disease in children, but they usually get ill in infancy. I know you're not ready to get tested, but when you are, I can do it here."

"I'm so afraid of people finding out."

"I promise you that no one will find out anything from this office about you or your husband." He added, "In the meantime, it might help you to talk to someone.

The radiation was finally ending and Mark was ready for us to return to Boston. The hospitals were more progressive and treatment for AIDS would be cutting edge. When we'd moved to Florida, we had rented out our south shore (Boston) house, which we had purchased after selling the house on the Vineyard, and the lease was up. Our small house in Florida could be sold.

An old college friend who knew that Mark had cancer and wanted to do something to help had contacted him about a job working with a group of high school-aged 'wanna be' pop stars. With his extensive teaching experience, Harvard degree, background in psychology and wide skill set, he'd be the tutor for the group. It required traveling, but the money and insurance benefits were exceptional. The job started in September and by then he'd have recovered from the treatments. There was no way to know what disease might assault him next.

Flooded with uncertainty and fueled with growing anger about what Mark had done, I wanted to finish out the fall semester in Florida and return to Boston around Christmas.

Unhappy with my decision not to return to Boston with him, Mark argued that I was behaving irrationally. The kids could start school in September and I could teach part time. He'd be in and out and his family was near if I needed help.

"I have more support here." I countered.

"And who do you have here? Your folks are a three hour drive away, Marsha is busy, Annie works, and Sam has his own life."

Exasperated, he continued in his broken voice, "This makes no sense. You wouldn't even have to work! I want to be with my children, and we have a place in Boston and you 'have more support here.' I can't believe you'd do this to us."

"Mark, I'm not going to Boston now."

"You're doing this to punish me for telling you the truth."

"I need to figure this all out."

"Figure what out? What are you talking about?"

"Us, this, this whole thing."

"If you haven't noticed, I am dying." His voice getting hoarser, he rumbled on, "I just want us to be together for as long as I have left."

"I know that," I hesitated, despising myself in that moment, "but, I have to find a way to live with this. It's not punishment."

"I thought we'd finished this."

"No, we have not finished this." I turned on him, angry now at his dismissal. "Actually, I'm not sure we ever started this. I don't even know who you are. You've apparently led a double life for years. And I may be dying too, because of you!"

That night, feeling better, Mark went out for a drink with a young colleague, Sam.

When he came home I was asleep. Since the chemo we'd been sleeping in separate beds, and I didn't hear him come in.

The dream came as I lay still. Footsteps tapped down the hall, heels clicking on the hardwood floor. Silently, the door handle turned, the door gradually opening. A man crossed the threshold, his quiet steps muffled by the thick rug beside the bed. He stood next to the bed. He held a long knife, his hands cleaved to the base of the weapon, the point of the dagger directed down to my breast. Motionless, I couldn't move to avoid the blade and before the cold steel touched my skin, the man stopped.

Waking, I screamed, my hair tangled in vines, twisted around my neck. Frantically, I jerked at the strands of damp hair in an effort to breathe.

Silhouetted in the shadows, Mark stood beside the bed. "Kathy, are you all right? I heard you scream."

"I'm all right, it was just a bad dream."

The following day, I sat with Dr. David Noble, who directed the local counseling center. I'd been seeing him weekly since Hal Jacobsen had mentioned it. His therapeutic style was to say little and have me process how I felt, a Gestalt, he interpreted. I loathed the whole process, but I liked David. I reluctantly related the recent dream, knowing about all about the symbolism, the phallic machete, the thrusting knife, the anonymous man, and my powerlessness.

David wanted me to finish the foolish dream. Talk it out and then 'feel it all'.

"But I may never have it again."

"It's okay if it never occurs again, but sometimes when we allow the dream to continue safely to the end, then the fear is diffused."

"We've already done this in the dream where I fell down into the water with the dead man." I frowned out the window. "I had that dream before I knew about Mark." I paused, "Another life ago."

David leaned forward. "Talk about what's happening right now with your body." He waited, then, when I said nothing, he went on, "What's your face doing right now? Your throat?"

"You know I hate doing this," I groaned. "You know my face looks sad."

"I know. I know you don't like it, but try to do it anyway."

I swallowed and breathed in, "My face feels like it's falling and my eyes are stinging a little bit. My throat is tight and it's hard to keep the words coming out. It hurts to swallow." Rolling my eyes, I continued, "Other than that I'm just fine."

"What else is going on? What's your breathing like?"

"Well, for now I'm breathing. As you can see, I'm still alive." I snidely said.

When David said nothing I sighed. "It's sort of constricted. If I take deep breaths it stops and catches."

"Good, now what if you let it go? Just let it all go. Stop fighting whatever your body is doing."

"I can't do that."

"Yes, you can."

I began to cry, slowly at first, then the tears quickened, and soon I was sobbing. "This is not okay, damn it! It's just not okay," I mumbled through the tears. "See, now are you happy? Is this what you want... me 'feeling'?"

He passed me the box of tissues. "I know you're angry and sad. It's what you need to get out. You function so much in your head and keep so much hidden. It's how you feel comfortable, but it won't work with this. If you don't look at and change patterns they're destined to repeat themselves."

"So, what now, you're Karl Marx?"

He smiled.

"Okay, you're right, you win." I paused and gulped in air. "I am in my head. It's how I've lived all these years. It's what I do. The heady part comes so easy for me. The gut stuff is hard and just sucks."

I wiped my eyes on the crumpled tissue and glared at him. "But, you know that, don't you. That's why you do this with me. It's why you push it."

"You know therapy is hard work and not always pleasant." He reached over for my hand. "You're going to get through this because you're strong. All I'm doing is providing a little guidance along the way." He stood up, the signal that the session was over. "Call me if you need me, otherwise, I'll see you next week."

Mark had returned to our house in Boston and was on his way back down to Florida to see me and the kids. He complained about our living situation and my upcoming plans.

"This whole timing of your visit is foolish. Olivia and Patricia will understand and I have to know when you and the kids are moving up. I've reserved a van to move furniture in early December," his voice crackled over the phone lines.

I was going to see my two close friends outside of Boston for a long weekend. As much as I dreaded it, I needed to let them know what was going on.

"I haven't seen them in a while and I need to tell them what's going on. They don't understand. They're our children's godmothers for heaven's sake! They deserve to know the truth. This way you can stay here with the kids. Jake's spending the night at Marsha's, and Lucy wants to ride to the airport with me."

"Who's driving you?"

"Sam. He'll stay with Lucy till you get home."

"I don't get in until late. That's a long time for Sam to have to keep Lu."

"He doesn't mind and she's elated. He's promised to teach her to dive."

Mark fumed. "The kids farmed out and you and me passing in the airport."

"I don't care how crazy you think it is," I shot back. "The plans are all set and I'm driving from Boston. I'll rent a car if you won't leave yours at the airport."

"Oh, for God's sake. I'll leave the car. You have keys. It just seems crazy, that's all."

I packed lightly and dropped Jake at Marsha's. I was writing Mark a note about food for the kids when I heard Sam pull into the driveway.

Lucy dashed down the hall and ran out the door just as Sam stepped out of the car.

"Well, hello, Lucy in the sky with diamonds." I watched him bend down to scoop Lucy up as she settled into Sam's amazing arms.

"I am Miss Lucy."

"Whoa, well, excuuuuse me, Miss Lucy in the sky."

"Oh," she wriggled down from his arms and took his hand, "I can't wait to dive. I can do it a little bit." She whispered, "Can we get Burger King on the way home? Can we, can we? Mom won't care."

"Yummy, Burger King. My fave." Pointing his finger in his open mouth he gagged and laughed as he took her hand and came into the house.

I waited by the door with my small suitcase ready to go. "Hi, I see she found you."

"Hey traveling lady," he nodded. "Looks like you're ready to hit the road?"

"Come on," Lucy whined pulling on my hand. "Let's go so we can get back and Sam can teach me to dive. I want to surprise Daddy."

I put my arm around her and laughed, "Well, no doubting what your priorities are!"

"I'll put this in the car and we'll get this show going." He took Lucy's hand, "Gotta hurry back to be ready for that diving competition."

"I can already dive a little, so I'll learn quick."

I got in the front seat beside Sam and Lucy climbed in the back. "You can have shotgun now, cause I get it on the way back."

"Well thanks, that was thoughtful of you," I grinned back at my daughter.

We drove without talking as Lucy softly hummed in the backseat. Soon the humming stopped, and I looked around to check on Lucy. She had fallen asleep.

I turned to Sam, "This is nice of you to take this time. She was so excited she was spending time with you, without Jake."

"She's a great kid and no trouble. It's the least I can do to help you all out."

"You've already done so much." Unbidden, he'd show up and take both children for ice cream, or a movie or just to go riding in his Jeep. I studied Sam's face as he drove. Handsome and young, he seemed older than his 26 years. He thrived in the Florida sun, his olive skin always tan and his dark, wavy hair flecked with red streaks. I had teased him about 'highlighting' it, and he had commented that it was his mother's genes coming out in his hair. About my height, he was stocky and powerful, had played baseball in college, full ride, until he damaged his knee and his trip to the majors flew out the window.

He glanced sideways and noticed me checking him out.

"I dressed for this, you know," he quipped. He wore his usual, a T-shirt, shorts and his proverbial footwear, flip flops. As he smiled I noticed the beginning of crow's feet crinkling around his eyes

"I figured. You always know how to impress the women."

"Well, I've impressed you," he countered.

"Ha, that's what you think, I just needed a ride," I laughed.

He grinned back, "It's good to hear you laugh. I don't hear it much anymore."

I avoided his eyes, "I know. It's been a lot to deal with."

"But, things are looking up. Mark's job is working out, he's over the chemo torture, and you all will be home in Boston by Christmas."

We rode in silence for a few moments.

"Hey, it's none of my business, and you can tell me to shut up, but you and Mark apart is weird. I understand you not wanting to let Marsha down, but she could find someone to take your place." He paused, "Well, of course no one would be you but," his voice trailed off.

"It isn't just that," I stared out the window.

Sam was quiet.

"I know it doesn't make any sense Sam."

He turned his head and looked directly at me. "I just can't see your not being with him. He's been so sick and you've been so worried all the time."

I looked away.

"Whatever's going on, it's between you guys, but I'm here if you need me. Whenever. Whatever you need."

I reached over and put my hand on his bare arm, "I know. Thank you."

"You're an incredible, strong woman." He grinned, scanning my bare knees, "And you got great legs."

"Well, as I've heard you previously declare, 'show me a tall, smart woman in a short skirt and you'd follow her anywhere'."

From the backseat came, "Hey, we there yet?"

"Almost, honey."

Chapter 6

Early fall in New England, the windows down in the car, I pulled over to the side of the road and got out inhaling the sweet aroma of the Rugosa roses which tumbled wild along the rocky jetty. The scene took me back to the summers we spent on this shore. Lucy had paddled around in the quiet waters, and I'd nursed Jake on the open porch as the waves rolled in.

Over a year had gone by since I'd been here and the beach was the same; a constant, like this fear I was living with. The sea storms came and the ocean raged, followed by a seductive calm, the foreboding always there, punctuated by the glorious respites. It seemed a fitting analogy to my current life, except the beach miraculously repaired itself.

Back in the car my head tilted back, eyes closed, face warm against the sun, I lingered in this in between space. Though Patricia and Olivia were two of my closest friends, I dreaded sharing the news. People were afraid, and then, never far away, lurking, poised for attack, the ominous villain, my own health. It was time people who loved me were told the truth. Time for me to face at least one of the fears I could control.

I started the car and wound down the road toward the house. In the circular driveway, I got out, and walked up the familiar path. With a lump in my throat I raised the polished brass knocker, opened the door and yelled, "I'm here, where are you?"

From the kitchen came Olivia's delighted shriek. She grabbed me in a fierce hug, going on about the lobster stew, the chilled wine, I was so thin and how late our dear Patricia was. Releasing me, she held my hand and propelled me into the kitchen.

"I haven't stopped talking and you haven't said a word. Oh, I'm just so happy you could come!" she gushed and handed me a glass of white wine.

"Me too. It's been too long. I've missed you guys so much!"

"How are you doing? Other than enviably thin?"

"Well, that's one good thing, but otherwise, I'm pretty awful. It's just wonderful to be away for a while and see you two." I took a sip of wine.

"But it's over for now and Mark's doing better. He's working at this new job. I spoke with him this morning, and he sounded okay." She offered, hopefully.

"He's not."

"But people get over this. They survive. Maybe the worst is over. You have to believe that, Kath."

I didn't respond.

Olivia continued on about psycho neuroanatomy stuff and thinking positive. It took all I had not to scream that no amount of positivity would cure AIDS! I gazed past Olivia at the early fall watercolor shades outside the leaded glass window, fingered the top of the wine glass and said nothing.

"C'mon," Olivia reached over the counter and touched my hand. "Let's go outside, while it's still warm and wait for her. She'll be faster if she thinks we're either, talking about her, drinking more wine, or planning dinner without her."

As we stepped over the threshold on to the terrace, I drew in a long breath. The roses on the wall perfumed the breeze and the earthy smell of the surrounding salt marshes punctuated the air. I'd forgotten the effect of the beauty of this place. And with it came dear Olivia. At just under six feet, she had a few inches on me, and carried the height regally. Wielding serious influence on a number of boards, she gave unflinchingly to a number of causes. Not able to have a biological child, she and her husband had adopted two children, one with a disability.

She caught me staring, turned to her and smiled. "We've had such wonderful times. Just the other day Steven reminded me that next summer you all are coming to the Cape for the Fourth."

I raised my eyebrows.

"I know that's far away, but you know us, we plan way ahead for that. The treatments and sickness will be behind you all, and we're going to celebrate."

Her voice trailed off as Patricia waltzed in. Everything about Patricia's movements were fluid. Moving about quickly was anathema to her. Not as tall as Olivia or I, with short wavy hair, she had the coloring of a true strawberry blonde with skin that stayed burnished peach all summer. Wearing simple khaki pants and a blue cotton sweater made her eyes appear even bluer.

"Oh my goodness, I'm so glad to see you," she butterfly kissed my cheeks. "How I've missed you, and you're finally here and everyone's left us alone. Isn't it incredible? And you're so thin. Well, I'm going to lose at least ten pounds soon. I love you both, even if you're richer and thinner than I'll ever be. And aren't we lucky to have each other. Sit down." She gestured to the chairs and settee.

Olivia tossed her head laughing, "Well, then of course we'll all sit down. She, who must be obeyed, has spoken!" and plopped down.

I grinned at both women and settled into the plump cushions of the settee next to Patricia.

"Now, stop being mean, to me," Patricia huffed at Olivia. "She has just gotten so bossy with you gone."

I grinned, thinking, thank goodness, some things never change.

"Well, we've missed you terribly. It's not the same without you. No one can take your place."

"Who'd want to?" giggled Olivia.

We all laughed.

"How's Mark and my precious god daughter?" asked Patricia.

"She's not just your god daughter," Olivia corrected. "You know we *both* said a vow."

"Lucy is great and she wanted to be sure I gave both her god mothers kisses from her." I paused, my face clouding over, not sure where to go with this. "Mark's doing all right considering what he's been through. The treatments are over for now. We'll have to wait and see."

"When are you and the kids coming back?" questioned Olivia. The conversation drifted to Mark's new job, his travel schedule, the stellar hospitals in Boston.

Finally, Patricia interrupted, "I still don't understand why you stayed in Florida."

When I didn't respond she went on, "We figured your parents are there and your job, I guess. Mark said you were coming in December when the semester was over."

I said nothing. Silence hung heavy over the porch.

Olivia said, "It's getting chilly, let's go back inside."

Inside, I sat at the counter, wondering how to begin when Patricia came from the butler's pantry carrying two glasses of wine.

She handed me a glass and sat down. "You know we just don't understand what you and Mark are doing apart. It doesn't make any sense."

Not meeting Patricia's eyes, I took a drink.

"I know it's nobody's business," Patricia put her hand on mine. "Whatever it is, you can work it out. I have faith in both of you."

I looked down into my wine. The worry never went away. "I thought being here in this place where the memories are so good and with you two here…" Overwhelmed by how to continue, tears welled up and spilled over running down my cheeks. "I'm scared and nothing seems to make it better."

Patricia put her arm around me, and I cried into her shoulder. Olivia walked over to the counter and sat down on my other side.

I lifted my head. "I have to tell you something. It's probably the hardest thing I've ever had to say, but I have to tell you." I wiped my eyes with the back of my hand. "It's more than cancer. Mark won't get well. He'll just get sick again."

"What are you talking about?" Olivia asked.

"Mark is HIV positive."

No one spoke. Olivia and Patricia stared at me, uncomprehending.

"Mark has the virus that causes AIDS. His cancer is a result of the virus."

"What?" Patricia asked, her eyes opening wide, shock evidenced on her face.

Shaking her head, Olivia sat forward, "I, I don't understand. Did he get it in the hospital? When did he get it? Has he had a transfusion? I thought the blood supply was safe. Oh, dear God." She covered her mouth with her hand.

With difficulty, I went on, "No, he didn't get it in the hospital. Blood supplies are safe."

"Well, good Lord, then how did he get it?"

"He got it through sex."

"Sex, sex with whom? What are you talking about?"

"All I know is what he told me. He told me that he's had sex with a number of people over the years, and he thinks he may have gotten it a year or so ago."

"So he doesn't have cancer?" Patricia asked, incredulous.

"He does have cancer, but they think it's result of the HIV."

"I don't understand."

"He has lymphoma but after it was diagnosed, they found he had the HIV virus in his system. The cancer was due to the breakdown in his immune system. The doctors told us both at the same time, right after his surgery."

"So you've this known for a while?" Olivia asked, puzzled.

"Yes," I hung my head. "But Mark lied to me about how he contracted it. He lied to the doctors and everyone."

"How could he lie to the doctors?" questioned Patricia.

"He said he must have gotten it before we got married, a long time ago. It didn't make sense, but he swore it was true, so I believed him and the doctors had no choice but to go along with his story."

I paused, looking at the two women, "He just told me the truth a couple of months ago."

"Whom did he have sex with?" Olivia stammered.

"I don't know," I shook my head. "I don't know that he knows."

"How could he not know who he had sex with?"

"He said he's been fooling around for years."

"But I thought AIDS was a gay disease," Olivia said.

"Well, not just homosexual men get it."

"Did he get it from a man?"

"I don't know." I closed my eyes.

"Why didn't you tell us?" Patricia asked.

"I was afraid," I answered, opening my eyes.

"What about you and the kids? Are you okay?"

"I can't get tested yet. I know the kids are all right, because the only way they could have gotten it would have been in utero. Mark doesn't think he had it then."

"How does he know? And God, how can you believe him? How do you know the kids are all right?" Patricia's voice rose as she reached forward and took a long swig of wine.

"They know a good bit about how you contract AIDS. The kids wouldn't be as old as they are and as healthy as they are if they had it. The only way they could have gotten it is from me."

"But how can you be sure?" Olivia moved off of the bar stool and crossed behind the counter.

"I have to believe that the children are fine, I couldn't go on if I didn't think that."

I glanced over at Olivia, who stood distant in the late afternoon shadows. "I have to believe that they are all right. And I really do, now, that I know about Mark, because of their ages and the time line."

"What about you?" Patricia turned to me.

"I don't know if I'm okay, but it doesn't make sense to get tested yet."

"Why?"

"The test could read negative and be wrong. It's more accurate if you wait about a year." I paused, "Besides, if I'm going to die, I don't want to know it."

"But Kath, you have to find out. You need to know."

"What can I do if I know?"

"But there are things you could do," Patricia hesitated. "There are some treatments."

"There are no treatments. You get sick and you suffer and then die. I don't want to know when that's coming."

"But if you have it," Patricia stopped.

"If I have it, what?"

"Well, if you have it, you should know."

"Why? I don't want to know," I argued, irritated, my eyes darting between the two women.

"But you should. I'm concerned about you and your children." injected Patricia.

I glared at her. "You sure you're not concerned about you, just being with me."

"Oh stop," Patricia ordered. "That's not true. It's a contagious, deadly disease that they don't know much about. Of course, I'm not afraid of being with you, but...I would want to know if you were infected. That is true."

From the corner of the room, Olivia cut in, "What she's saying is that you need to know and we need to know, so we can help you."

"Help me do what?" I took a gulp of wine and slammed it down on the counter. "Help me? I think that's a load of crap. You just moved away from me. You want to know if you need to wash the glasses in Clorox and disinfect your clothes where I cried on you."

"No, that's not it," Patricia shut her eyes and shook her head.

"I can tell by the way you're both looking at me. You're afraid and aren't sure what to do with me."

"That's not true," Olivia's quiet voice came across the room.

"What is true then, dammit?" I fired back. "You got up and moved. You're horrified. You're shocked that this disease could possibly enter your pristine, ordered little world. My God, you actually know someone with AIDS. Your best friend might even have it. Even when I get tested you won't believe that I'm not contagious." I covered my face with my hands. The tears coursed down.

"I'm not scared of you," Patricia responded evenly. "But I am horrified. Not because I know someone with AIDS. I'm horrified at what I've just heard. Horrified at what Mark's done. I want to know if you're okay, because I love you and care about you. I know I won't get it by being with you. But, yes, I do want to know because I probably would be more cautious if I knew you had AIDS. That may be awful, unfair and not Christian, but it's how I feel."

Patricia glanced over at Olivia, who stood apart watching us.

I felt like a leper.

Olivia spoke, her voice trembling, "To be honest, I am concerned. I don't know much about the disease. Just what I hear on the news and see in magazines." She came over and sat down. "I feel awful even saying that. It sounds terrible, it makes me feel terrible, but it's the truth. I know what they say in the news, about it being hard to contract, but there's so much they don't know." She stopped and took a deep breath. "What if you cut yourself here? What would I do? How could I take care of you? I know that my life is sheltered and predictable, and I don't have a lot of experiences beyond all of this." She waved her hand around the room.

Patricia took my hand, her eyes tearing up. "I don't know what to think or what to do."

Olivia reached out and rested her hand on my knee. "Me either. I just want you and the kids to be all right."

Silence filled the room, the only sounds the quiet humming of the refrigerator in the distance.

"I'd never let anyone risk themselves taking care of me. They know you can't get it through drinking glasses, or crying on each other, or bodily contact.

I just have to believe I'm probably all right, given the time line. The few times Mark and I had sex after Jake was born, he used a condom." Smiling sadly, I continued, "That should have been a clue for me, but we'd used them before, so I didn't put it all together." I paused, "Anyhow, I will get tested. I want to wait until late fall, because that will be about a year from when I last had sex with Mark. The longer you wait, the more reliable the test. The doctor at home said I could do it in his office. I don't want anyone to know I'm even getting tested."

"People are scared of it all." Olivia gazed out the darkened window.

I looked at Olivia's lovely profile and then over at Patricia. "I know I have to be ready for the results, whatever they are. Right now, I'm hopeful and go on with that hope. If the test is positive for HIV then where is my hope?" *What do I do then?*

Chapter 7

Expecting the children, I was surprised to see only Sam waiting for me when I exited the plane. He smiled, chatted and took my bag as we began walking down the airport corridor.

I acted interested in his banter, smiled back and offered little information about the difficult trip. Then, I asked about the kids. Sam stared at me puzzled. They were at home with Mark. My mouth set in a straight line, I stalked on ahead of Sam.

"Hey, wait up," he gently grabbed my arm. "I ain't the porter."

I knew this had nothing to do with him. I stopped and turned, "I'm sorry, Sam. It's just that I didn't know Mark was home."

"Look, Kath. It is none of my business what's going on with you two, but your kids are thrilled that their dad is home."

"I know."

"Whatever it is, you love each other and have been through a rough time." He put his hand on my shoulder. "He's still hurting from all the treatments and seems pretty tired."

"It's complicated, Sam." We walked on not talking until we reached the car.

I got in and faced Sam. He deserved an answer of some kind. "I know you think I'm crazy to still be here when Mark is somewhere else, but it's what I have to do for now. I know everyone is probably talking about how selfish I'm being and wondering what the hell is going on."

Sam took my hand. "Whatever people think doesn't matter. I know you, and I know that you must have a damned good reason for doing what you're doing."

"Thank you." I felt the lump in my throat as the tears welled up.

Sam began to pull his T shirt off over his head, "Baby, I'm giving you the shirt off my back to wipe up your tears."

A weak smile played at the corners of my mouth. "Stop." I put my hand on his arm. "I know, you want me to see your chest, which is huge, as you've told me time and again."

"You got that right. Not as big as the doc's but still huge!" He bent his head over his shoulder and kissed each bicep with a loud smacking noise.

"You are such an ass."

"Ah, the goddess of perspicacity. And I can use big words too." He grinned over at me.

I laughed.

He started the car, and we began the journey home.

When we arrived home it was late, but the children were still awake and sitting with Mark watching TV. Jake ran to my outstretched arms. I hugged him close and blew a kiss to Lucy, who was transfixed by the television show and curled up on the sofa next to her dad.

I put Jake down and turned to Mark expressing my surprise that he was still here.

Not moving from the sofa, Mark nodded to Sam, "Hi." He shot me a sidelong glance. "Good to see you too." He continued, "As you can see, I am still here. The trip got cancelled so I'm home for a couple of more days. How was Boston?"

"It was fine. The car worked out well." I was barely holding it together when Sam put down a toy he had been fidgeting with and started towards the door. "I'll be on my way."

"Thanks for picking her up."

"Oh," I turned to Sam. "I'm sorry, thanks for the ride and the company."

"Bye, Sam," Lucy's voice emerged from the pillows. "I showed Daddy my dive but then it got cold."

"Good one Lu. You got it down."

From the floor in front of the TV came, "Bye, Sam." Twisting around, Jake held up his palm in a high five. "Later, dude," he commented in a near perfect Ninja Turtle imitation.

"Goodbye all," Sam said and let himself out.

I picked up my bag from the floor. No one followed as I walked down the hall and into the bedroom.

Putting the children to bed, after stories and kisses, they fell asleep. My hair still wet from the shower, I had slipped on my nightgown, when I heard voices coming from the living room. I tiptoed down the hall, saw Sam talking to Mark and hid in the dark hall eavesdropping.

"I don't understand this at all," Sam said. "Did you leave her or did she leave you?"

"No one has left anyone. We're apart for now and that's it."

"Hey, this is me, Sam. You can bullshit other people, but I want to know what's going on here."

"It's none of your business, really." Mark answered.

"It is my business. I'm a close friend and I want to help. It's obvious, something is wrong, you all are struggling."

Ignoring Sam's comment, Mark asked, "Want a beer?" and the men moved from the living room into the kitchen.

The voices got quiet, and I couldn't hear what they were saying, so I crept closer to the end of the hallway, hidden in the shadows.

Suddenly, Sam erupted, "How could you do that to her?"

I came out of the dark hall and looked from one to the other, "What's going on?"

Sam pointed at me. "Her, and your kids." He glared at Mark. "What the hell?"

I hung at the edge of the room, not moving.

The now empty beer bottle in his hand, Sam crossed in front of me and disappeared into the living room. Mark followed.

The front door slammed and then a thud as something banged against the side of the house. Entering the hall, I stopped abruptly as the door flew open, and Sam tore back in.

He faced Mark, his right hand tight around the neck of the empty bottle. "How in the name of God, could you have done what you did to your family?" He gestured at me. "I love her. I love her and I love your children." Swinging the empty bottle swung back and forth, he frowned disgustedly down at Mark who sat on the edge of the sofa, head in hand, his elbow propped on the sofa arm.

"If you're going to hit me with that bottle let me know. I bleed easily now." Mark muttered.

"You worthless bastard," Sam flung at Mark. He shook his head, "I want to hit you. I really do, but I won't. It's too easy."

I went over to Sam and put my hand out to touch him. He jerked away, startled, staring at me like he saw me there in the room for the first time.

"I'm leaving now." The bottle clattered to the floor.

"Sam..."

"I know the way out." He headed to the door, jerked it open and slammed out.

I whirled on Mark. "So, you told him the truth."

"Yes."

"Why?"

"He knew something was wrong with this whole charade of you keeping us apart. Sam knows us well. He knows we would never be apart if things were all right."

"Why did he come back?"

"I don't know. Maybe just to talk. We have been friends."

"What did you tell him?"

"That I was HIV positive."

"And about us, me and the kids?"

"He wanted to know."

"And what did you say?"

"For fuck's sake, I told him you and the kids were probably fine."

I bit my lip, saying nothing. Then, decisive, I went on, "Other people need to know the truth. At work, they think I'm a monster for abandoning you. Even my parents think I've lost it. "

Mark injected, "I thought we agreed not to say anything. People are still scared of this."

"They are. Even Olivia and Patricia were. I'm not saying we need to broadcast it, but people like Annie and Sam are our friends and they don't understand what we are doing apart."

"Well, I don't either."

"I'm sick of people thinking I'm the bad guy," I retorted.

"So, is that what I am now? The bad guy."

I didn't answer him. "Olivia and Patricia were wonderful when we finally got through it all. It was hard, but in the end it turned out okay." I paused, thinking out loud, "I'll tell my folks after I get tested, once I know something."

Reaching over and touching my knee, Mark implored, his tired eyes seeking mine, "Don't you know I feel terrible about what I've done? I'll do anything to make it up to you if you'd only give me a chance."

I jerked my leg back away from his touch. "I don't know what a chance is Mark, but I do know there are some things that can't be made up." I turned on him, "I'm going to bed. It's been a long day." In the bedroom, I closed the door and for the first time in the room alone, I locked it.

By late October, fall had arrived in central Florida, the weather changed, the days less humid, the nights crisp. Sam had more or less disappeared. I had seen him at work where he visited briefly. He was cordial and moved on. He'd taken Lucy swimming a few times, dropped her off and not come in. I tried to talk with him, but he wouldn't engage for any length of time.

Marsha told me that Sam was blown away by the news. In some way, he had idealized Mark and the truth devastated him. She said he'd come around in his own time.

Nightly, Mark phoned to talk with the children but hadn't been down all month. He'd been on the road with the group, who were banking huge amounts of publicity and becoming well known. He seemed to have little time, but would be here for Halloween.

Costume decisions were huge. Jake had to be a Ninja but couldn't decide if he wanted a turtle shell; Lucy, a Carebear, like her beloved bear Melvin, but the costume was troublesome. Unhappy with just bear ears and Carebear pajamas she debated changing to a pirate. Both children wanted their dad to see them and go trick or treating. Mark promised he'd be there for Halloween.

That night after tucking the children in bed, I fell into a troubled sleep. I'd been having the 'man with the knife' dream again, and the Xanax was not working. I was a hot mess. Waking up, sweating and fearful, I heard a noise. Eyes open in the muted light, I listened. The footfall, too heavy to be a child, stopped outside my closed door. I was awake, this was not a dream. Daring to breathe, I watched as the doorknob turned and someone entered the room. Approaching the bed, a man stood over me, just like in my dream. I screamed and rolled away.

"It's okay. It's just me." He switched on the light and I saw Mark's face.

A Red Door

Having heard the scream, the children dashed into the room. Lucy ran to her father's arms, and Jake backed away from his dad when he saw my face. "What happened to Mommy?" he climbed on the bed.

"Nothing, buddy. Mom's all right. I guess I scared her that's all. My plane got in early, and I came on home."

I had Jake in my arms. "Jake, honey, I'm okay. I just got scared." I turned to Mark. "Why didn't you call?"

"I don't know. It was late."

"Well, Daddy, you're here for Halloween, just like you promised," Lucy added. "Come see my costume, I'm a pirate."

Mark smiled at her and picked her up. "Miss Pirate, it's time for bed. We'll do costumes tomorrow. I believe you have school." He left the bedroom, carrying Lucy.

Jake stayed next to me. "Are you still scared Mommy? Cause if you are, I'll stay and protect you. I know all the Ninja stuff."

"No, sweetie, it's okay, Daddy's home, let's go to your bed. I'm fine. I'm not scared anymore, but I know you are one brave Ninja."

The next day I had an appointment with David and reported that the Xanax was not working. He suggested I needed something less addictive and would talk to Hal.

"Have you been having the machete dream as frequently?" David asked.

"No, not really, not since you made me finish it. I've only had it a few times and it's been months. Last night was different."

"What happened last night?"

I told him about Mark and waking up with him standing over me.

"Take his key."

"David, it's his house too. Mark wouldn't hurt us. He loves his children. And, I think he still loves me."

Eyebrows raised, David gently shook his head.

"I know, I know, how could he love us and do what he did? But I know he does love us in his own confused way."

"He will continue to do what he wants until you make him stop. A man whose actions risked his family's health will stop at nothing. He has few limits."

"David," I frowned, leaning forward in the chair. "He really does love his kids." I paused, "And, he's dying."

"As you said, the man played Russian Roulette with your lives. Those are your words." He stopped, letting the statement sink in. "He knew the risks. I'm not concerned about the reasons behind his behavior. That's for him and whomever he's seeing to figure out, if he's seeing anyone. I'm concerned about you."

"I can't keep him from seeing his kids."

"I realize he needs to see the children, but I see the effect his visits have on you. I see you begin to crawl out of the hole, and then fall back down when he comes and goes out of yours and the kids' lives."

"What would you have me do? Not let him see his children?"

"No. Your not going with him was psychologically healthy. It took you months of gut wrenching decision making, but it was the healthy thing to do. You came to it on your own. You are strong, a survivor and one of the sanest women I know." He stopped, his gaze holding my eyes, the purposeful silence punctuated only by the faint ticking of the wall clock.

"I see what he does to you, emotionally."

I said nothing, my eyes wandering out the upstairs window.

"Be cautious and set firm limits with him. I don't think you should be alone with him. Get legal if you have to. I believe you will eventually have to, because he hasn't proven reliable with money for the kids."

I glanced back at David when he mentioned money. I knew he was right, but it was so difficult to reconcile all of this with the man whom I had married.

"You said money was tight, and I know Mark makes plenty. I figured he was jerking you around with money. It's one way he has control."

"He forgets to pay the nursery school and the preschool teacher who takes care of the kids. I've told him that I'd take care of it if he just gave me the money." I paused, "But, he paid them on time this month."

"I believe that he is doing what he's always done, only now he's dying and has nothing to lose."

"David," Taking in what he was really saying, I shook my head, "You can't believe that Mark is still out there having sex and infecting others. I can't believe you're saying that."

"That's exactly what I'm saying," David commented, evenly.

"He wouldn't do that."

"I don't believe that behavior like Mark's goes away."

"Well, I can't believe that," I fiddled with my loose hair, avoiding David's gaze. "He's not amoral."

"I don't know. To risk your lives like he did requires a certain level of amorality. He somehow felt he was invincible. Mark's smart, charming, and I imagine he never thought about being caught."

"Well, he may be all of that, but I'm not ready to believe that he's still having sex and doesn't feel remorse for what he's done."

"Oh, I think he does feel remorse," David replied, with a nod. "I just wonder if the remorse is that he got caught." He paused, glanced away from me and then continued, "Maybe not, maybe I'm wrong. Just be careful and set some limits with him."

Chapter 8

Following David's disturbing analysis, I drove home in a funk. I wanted to avoid Mark, but he was staying through the Halloween weekend to take the kids out for trick or treat. Lucy, finally deciding on a patched eye pirate and Jake, in Ninja garb complete with turtle shell were thrilled that Daddy would take them around the neighborhood.

Since Mark had taken on the trick or treat responsibility, Marsha and I decided to have dinner at our favorite Mexican place. We met at Marsha's house, going in one car.

A few shots of tequila later, I knew I wouldn't be driving. I phoned home to let Mark know and Loren, our favorite babysitter answered. Mark had called her and gone out after the Halloween festivities had died down.

"He said he'd be late so not to worry. He thought you'd be home before he got here."

"Hmm, well." I mumbled through the tequila haze, guilt saturating every pore. "I'm at Dr. Glines' and am spending the night, so I won't be home until tomorrow."

Loren assured me she was okay and figured Mark would be home soon. The kids were wiped out and dead asleep.

Not showering or even brushing my teeth, I fell into an alcohol induced slumber. No dreams of men with machetes or anything I could remember, I woke up the next morning, my mouth cotton and my head ringing. Before I could get out of bed, Marsha appeared with a glass of ginger ale and two aspirins.

"Here, take, swallow and don't speak. I didn't drink half of what you did, but I feel like I've been run over with a mower, and my mouth feels like the bottom of a bird cage."

"That's so poetic."

"I said, don't speak." She wheeled around and left the room as I swallowed the aspirin.

Getting up required supreme effort and reminded me why I should not drink tequila. Carefully, I washed my face, swished toothpaste in my mouth and reluctantly, put on my rumpled clothes from the night before.

In the kitchen, Marsha stood silently by the coffee maker.

I draped my arm around her shoulder. "Well, you didn't drink as much as I did?"

"No, but I drank too much. You drank an obscene amount. I was waiting for you to lose it."

"Thank the Lord, I never did. I just passed out."

"I thought we'd been there, done that. I'm way too old for a hangover." Marsha rubbed her temples. "God, I have a headache."

"Where are Ron and the girls?"

"Ron took one look at me and whisked the girls off to breakfast. It's Saturday, remember?"

I slid down in the chair feeling awful. Marsha handed me a mug of coffee.

"I need to get home." I remembered calling home and Loren was there.

Marsha handed me a slice of warm toast. "It will soak up the alcohol."

"I don't think I can eat anything."

"Don't argue. Eat it."

I screwed up my face and mouthed the dry toast, while Marsha reminded me again that we were way too old for this.

"You're telling me. When we were twenty, hangovers were a walk in the park and now I can hardly even stand up. I feel horrible. I have to get home."

"Have another cup of coffee and you'll feel better."

I finished the second cup of coffee and drove home, surprised to see Loren's car in the driveway. It seems that she was asleep when Mark got home so she'd stayed the night. She hadn't seen him, but the kids said he was in bed. It was all fine, she reiterated. Jake was next door until after lunch, and Lucy was in the back watching TV. Loren had been concerned about taking care of the children. I asked her what time had Mark gotten home.

"Well," Loren hesitated. "He went out about nine and I don't really know, maybe sometime after 2:00. I fell asleep on the couch after the late movie."

"Loren, he got home at two in the morning?"

Loren nodded, uncomfortable. "Well, I was asleep so I just stayed. I wanted to be here if the kids woke up."

I hugged her and apologized again. Reaching into my purse, I grabbed a wad of cash.

Loren smiled, "That's too much. It's not like I had a hot date or anything. Lucy and Jake are like my family. I'd never want them to be scared or worried. It's really okay."

"No, it's not okay, Loren. I am awfully sorry this happened."

After Loren left, I looked in on Lucy, who was flopped out on the floor absorbed in a cartoon. I ignored the door to the spare room where Mark slept. Shrugging out of my dirty clothes, I hopped in the shower, dried off and slapped on a bit of makeup hoping to hide the hangover pallor. Peering in the mirror, I realized it didn't help. The day would be a washout. Maybe by afternoon, I'd have recovered. I got a Coke and carried it out to the porch where I switched on the overhead fan and eased down in the large wicker chair. Holding the cold glass to my throbbing head, I closed my eyes and didn't hear Mark come out to the porch.

"Tequila has never been your friend," he sat down on the chair across from me.

I lowered the dripping glass. "Where were you until the wee hours? Loren was still here when I got home."

"I went out."

"That's obvious. Loren stayed over."

"Look, I thought you would be home, not out drinking too much. You weren't. Loren was fine."

I leaned forward in the chair, "Mark, what the hell were you doing until 2:00 AM?"

"It wasn't 2:00. I got home late and Loren was asleep. I didn't wake her." He glared at me and got up. "I'm leaving Sunday, so I planned to take the kids to the movies today." He moved to the door. "I'll feed them an early dinner somewhere. I don't imagine you want to come."

"No, I don't want to come."

A Red Door

Alone on the porch, I thought about what David had said. What was Mark doing out all that time? I got up and went to the kitchen phone to dial Loren's number. I needed to find out if I was losing it.

"Hey, it's me. Quick question, did you say Mark got home after 2:00?"

"Yeah, it was about then. I remember cause the late movie got over right around 2:00. I looked at the clock when I got a blanket out of the closet." She waffled, "I was okay, really. It's not a big deal, he's stayed late before when I've been there."

"He stayed out that late before?"

"Uh huh. When you've been out of town. He told me he was going into Orlando and he'd be late."

I hung up the phone and stood there, dumbfounded, looking out the window at Mark pushing Lucy in the swing. The man I'd married, a good dad who loves his kids but who had risked their lives by his pattern of behavior. It made no sense. Could David be right? Was Mark, no longer visibly ill, back to what he did before? I leaned my head on the refrigerator hoping for some enlightenment as to why. Resting there with the tears seeping out, I wondered if anything had changed for him.

The next day, even though I knew we should talk, I avoided Mark. He knew it too and ignored me when I was around. Sam appeared to have disappeared. All he told Marsha was he needed to take off for a few days and had his classes covered. He hadn't mentioned where he was going.

Finally, Mark headed back to Boston and life fell back into the routine we'd established. Lucy moped around for a day or two after he left but then got back into school and her friends. Jake, unaffected by the coming and going was his usual cheerful, energetic self. Annie and her little boy, who was Jake's age, were coming for the weekend.

Annie dropped down in the chair on the porch, dropping her oversized bag by the wall. "I don't know how you do it." She tossed her tousled short, dark brown curls. "I mean the two kids and all, by yourself."

"I drink. Daily. It's past 5:00. Red or white?"

"When we're old and go to the home we have to find one that celebrates happy hour."

"By then, I figure we won't know or care if it's 5:00."

We sat in comfortable silence drinking wine for a few moments. I looked over at Annie. She was my oldest friend; we'd met as babies in the church nursery when I bit her. Funny thing is that Jake bit her baby boy too (we must have some biting gene), and she still loved us. When teenagers, we'd traded clothes, smoked our first cigarettes, sneaked out together and cried over lost boyfriends. Annie, a bit taller than I was, was an athlete in high school. Wearing her uniform of short shorts and an Ann Taylor tee, into her late thirties, she had the fit body of a college swimmer.

When Mark and I moved to Florida, we resumed the friendship that had endured through the many years of living far apart. Annie was divorced and lived where we grew up, about 3 hours away. Jake and her son were the same age, we were even pregnant at the same time, and had become compatible playmates.

I knew it was time to tell her the truth when she asked how I was really doing without Mark.

"Without Mark," I repeated Annie's words. "Oh, honey, it's such a mess. It's not what it seems."

"Well, who cares what it seems. Most things aren't. Whatever it is won't change anything. You could never do anything to change us."

"Oh, Lord!" I grinned, finally imagining what folks must think. "I'm not having an affair or anything tawdry like that. I only wish." I swallowed and barreled on. "It's Mark. He's HIV positive. He has the virus that causes AIDS. The cancer was a result of the HIV infection."

Annie reached out and grabbed my hand not saying anything. Slowly, she let go, stood up and put her arms around me.

"And you and the kids are all right?" she asked softly.

"I don't know," I answered. "The kids are probably okay. If they had it, at their ages they'd be sick. Me, I don't know yet."

She went back to the chair and sat down. Leaning forward she took a gulp of wine. "I've got to have a ciggy." She got up, found her bag and rummaged around until she found cigarettes and a lighter. Her hand shaking, she lit the cigarette and took a long drag. "I know you hate me smoking, but we're on the porch."

"I do, but it's okay. You'll need more before I finish this sordid tale." I said with a weak grin. " I have to wait to get tested because the test can be false negative if I don't wait long enough."

"You don't have AIDS. You're fine."

"Some days I really believe that and then I think after all this time, how could I have escaped?"

"You do not have AIDS. I know you don't."

"Oh, Annie, you love me and can't imagine I'd be ill, and I love you too."

"That's true," she paused, taking another puff, "but you don't have it." She shook her head and shrugged her shoulders as if to say 'that's that'.

I related the wretched story as I knew it, including Mark's confession.

"Good God! He's just been screwing around with whomever."

"From what he told me," I hesitated, "it's been going on for a while."

"Good Lord in heaven, it's a good thing he's not here. I'd like to ring his scrawny neck." She paused, "So what about the cancer?"

"Oh, he has cancer but like I said, it's a result of the HIV."

"I didn't hear much after you said HIV." She gazed at me and took a long drag. "I may need more ciggies and wine." Sighing, she asked, "Have you told your folks?"

"No, I can't until I know whether I'm okay. Once I know, good or bad, I'll tell them."

"But you are okay. You are. So, who else knows about all this?"

"Just Marsha, Sam, as of the other day, Olivia and Patricia, Mark's brother and some of the doctors. Sam stormed out and almost hit Mark when he found out. He's not at work and seems to have vanished. I've been afraid to tell because of the stigma and the kids. It's a small town and people are so freaked out and scared about the disease. Mark's brother, bless him, calls almost daily to check on me and the kids. And Mark has close friends in Boston, which is a good thing. It is better he's there."

"It is. This place is so backward. They burned down the house that belonged to that family whose kids had AIDS. Thank God, they had moved out."

Noises erupted as Jake and Lucy came running onto the porch, shrieking. Lucy had her hands on her hips and stamped her feet as Jake gloated and ducked behind Annie's chair. Fighting had ensued over Melvin, Lucy's beloved Carebear.

"He stole Melvin! Make him give it back!" Lucy demanded.

Annie got up and took Lucy's hand. "I have an idea. You can spend the night in my room, and we can play Carebears tonight. And I bet by the time, Melvin will be rescued."

All finally settled down, and I was in the kitchen ferreting through the pantry. I turned around and there was Annie. She took me in her arms, tears filling her expressive brown eyes, "You have been in my life since you bit me in the nursery and left a welt on my sweet cheek and I'm not about to lose you now. The good Lord won't let that happen. It's not your time," she smiled through the tears, "we have too much to do as yet." Standing still in the kitchen, we held on tightly as the dappled light faded into dusk.

That night Jake slipped into my bed when I was in the shower. When I came out he had covered his head and was snuggled down under the comforter. I laughed and climbed into bed patting the lump next to me.

"Well, what can this big pillow be? Maybe if I tickle it, it will move over."

"Noooo, no tickles, it's just me, Jake." Jake popped his head out from the covers. "Can I stay here? I'll keep the scary dreams away."

"My brave Ninja. I guess so. For tonight. We'll keep each other company."

I kissed him on the forehead and turned out the light.

The weekend passed and Monday came and went. Tuesday brought another sleep troubled night. Then it came to me, I had this idea (it was probably the drugs), that if I could exorcise the demons who frolicked in my bed and tormented me with god awful dreams, I might begin to sleep again, unassisted by pharmaceuticals.

You know when you are in the middle of doing something that you realize is kind of crazy, but you do it anyway. That's the way it was that morning. After dropping the children at school, I came home and in a fit, ripped the covers off our bed, dragged them outside to the backyard and threw them in a heap. I marched into the storage room and got the lighter fluid, poured it all over the pile of bed stuff, lit a match and watched as the funeral pyre reduced these representations of the life I'd lost to smoldering rubble. Seeing it sputter and finally catch on with that whoosh fire makes, I bit my lip and my eyes started to smart, tears mingling with the salty perspiration. I got sad thinking about the long gone, lovemaking those linens had hosted. The tentative beginnings, the quiet slow build up, the gradual glow as you teeter there, close to blazing. Then, finally, gratefully, you give in, the fire spent and like the dying embers, you rest there, released.

That night, once again, sleepless, not at all released, I lay like a forgotten missive, folded between the pages of new, crisp sheets. In the silvery half-light of a fading Florida evening, the bat winged water stain, Rorschached on the bedroom ceiling hovered. Fitful, I wondered if I'd ever make love with anyone, again? Could I claim virginal status since I hadn't had sex for almost a year? 'Virgin again' is an oxymoron, but maybe if you'd been celibate for a while you could declare yourself born again. Rebirth was possible if the right person came along, but in the meanwhile, it had been a long time.

I switched on the bedside lamp and sat up in bed. In the night table drawer the 'virgin' vibrator lay in its narrow, innocuous box tucked in the back beside the Mace. I purposely kept it in the box because I thought if I decided to use it I could see myself groping in the dark and using the Mace instead of the 'eight ridged inches' promised to 'light up my life'.

The vibrator had been a joke gift for my thirty seventh birthday. My romantic self, laughed that it was so contrived, not at all sensuous.

Annie had countered with, "You want romance, light a candle! Of course it's not sensuous. It just feels good and sometimes this works just fine."

How times had changed.

I slid the vibrator out of the box and smiled at its ridiculous imitation of a penis, long and stiff, with ridges around the shaft. Rotating the base around to turn it on nothing happened, no vibration, no light. I shook it and tried to turn it on again, then realized that the batteries were dead.

This was no good; then I remembered I had just put new size 2D batteries in Jake's robot, so I slid out of bed and tiptoed quietly down the hall into his room. Sidling over to the bed, I peered at my sleeping child. As my eyes adjusted to the dark, I crept around cautiously avoiding the multitude of toys littering the floor, praying my child wouldn't wake up. I spotted the robot beside his bed. Carefully, picking it up, I scurried back to my room. Removing the robot's base, I took out the batteries and put them into the vibrator. I turned the vibrator on, the tip lit up and the object began to gently quiver.

I placed the impotent robot on the floor, closed the bedroom door and climbed into bed. I turned out the light and the soft glow from the moving vibrator lit up the area around it, just like the box promised. The penis pulsated. I burst out laughing with visions of immobile, silent toys in puzzled children's rooms; robots whose arms wouldn't work, dogs that didn't yip and cars that couldn't go, frustrated children with their paralyzed toys whining, while the moms' serenely smiled and bought batteries in bulk.

Putting the 'light up my life' under the covers I closed my eyes.

Chapter 9

The idea of Mark still being out there, maybe infecting others, made me crazy. It seemed impossible, but then again, what happened to us seemed impossible. Concentrating on anything for long was a challenge.

And I missed Sam. He was usually such a good sounding board when I was stewing about something. I stopped by his empty office and left him a note. Surely, he would come around soon.

At lunch with Marsha, I told her about Mark staying out, and the troubling issue David had raised.

"You know, I trust David completely. That's why I suggested you see him. He's so damned intuitive, in addition to being a skilled therapist. It's what makes him good,"

"But, Marsh you know Mark. You're fond of Mark. Can you see him, sexually active, given his diagnosis?"

"No, but I couldn't see him doing what he did to you all either."

We ate in silence for a few moments before Marsha raised the issue of me getting tested.

I didn't answer right away and looked down fiddling with my food.

"Well, is the salad finally stirred up enough?" Marsha grinned over at me.

I sighed, smiling back, "It's hard to believe it's been almost a year since I probably would have been infected. Actually, since I've had sex. That is, sex with a person."

Marsha laughed. She knew about the vibrator and borrowed batteries. Continuing on a serious note, she suggested given the length of time, I could find out and go from there.

I stretched across the table, my voice low, "Yes, if it's negative, but what if it isn't? Then, I know it's just a matter of time."

"No," Marsha emphasized in her most business like voice. "Then you go to Boston and get into an experimental program and live as long as you can for your kids." She reached out and put her hand on mine. "You're living now like you have it. You cover it well, but I know you. You hardly eat, you don't sleep, you're anxious, and the last time you had a cold you freaked."

My eyes swept down to the table. "Is it that obvious?"

"To me. I've known you for a long time and I see you almost every day." She looked hard at me. "How much worse off can you be? And you may not have it."

Resting my chin in my hand, elbow on the table, I shut my eyes and breathed deeply. *Dear God, it would be so wonderful to wake up and not worry that I could be sick. Every day at some point it comes to me. It hits me at odd moments. I'll be getting Jake dressed and think about it or I'll be making supper or sitting in my office.* After a moment I opened my eyes. "You're right. If I have it how much worse off can I be?"

"And you know that whatever the outcome, I'll be there, no matter what."

The week after my conversation with Marsha, I called Hal Jacobsen's office and went alone, not telling anyone. His receptionist recognized me and told him I had arrived. Late in the day, no one remained in the waiting room. Dr. Jacobsen came out immediately and took me into his office.

I thanked him for seeing me without a real appointment. They only saw patients till lunch on that day so I was in luck. We talked for a few minutes about my sleeping, general health, then I knew it was time. I took the leap.

"Okay. I'm here and I need you to do the test right now before I change my mind? It's been about a year. Can you do it and not let anyone know?"

He waited a moment. "Of course. I told you I would when you were ready." He explained that he'd draw my blood and run it as a Jane K. Smith and then do his own, and they'll both be labeled Jane Smith, his with a different middle initial.

I stammered and swallowed hard, the familiar lump building in my throat.

"I have to tell you, you've got to come back in person for the results. I won't do it over the phone. You can wait as long as you need to until you feel you can hear the results, then, you call me when you are ready. Then, you come in."

I nodded, tears in my eyes. I had to do this. I didn't want to live the way I was anymore, and I needed to know, not matter the outcome.

"Whatever the outcome, I'll be there and help you cope with it. It's been about ten months since Mark was diagnosed and longer since you would have been infected. Right?"

Nodding, I bit my lip, my face pale. "I think so."

He took my hand, smiling gently. "I've seen you go through a lot already. You're strong. You can do this and I admire you. I want you to know that."

"Thank you. I don't feel any of that right now, just really scared. So let's get on with this before I chicken out."

He got up and led me down the hall to one of the examining rooms. I sat on the table, my face to the wall, eyes squeezed shut as my arm trembled. He put the elastic band on my arm and I made a fist. The needle pricked and the tears that I'd been holding back dripped into my mouth. He filled two test tubes, gave me a cotton ball to hold to my arm and told me he'd be right back as he left the room.

I sat pressing the cotton to my arm when a nurse came in.

"Oh, I didn't know anyone was in here." Puzzled, she looked at the test tubes. "I should label those before they get misplaced." Walking over to the tubes she took out her pen to write on the label. "Remind me of your name?"

I stared at her.

"Your name, honey?"

At that moment Hal swung open the door. "I'll take that." He reached over and took the tube out of the nurse's hand.

Surprised, she responded, "I was just labeling the samples."

"I can do it myself, thanks."

"But Dr. Jacobsen, I usually do that."

"Thanks, but it's late, go home. I'll finish up here." He shooed her out of the door and closed it behind her.

"Now, she'll be curious about me."

"Good, we'll be gossip for her. Give her something to wonder about."

I shot him a weak smile. "Dr. Jacobsen, thank you so much for doing this. You made it as painless as it could have been."

"It's something I can do. One favor please, just call me Hal."

I studied this kind man with pale blue eyes above a reddish beard. He was a little taller than I, someone you wouldn't look at twice if you passed on the street. His quiet voice exuded calm. His hands were large, with clipped immaculate nails, no ring. There was a small hole in his ear where it had once been pierced. I knew nothing about him except where he went to med school, and he knew all the messy, seamy details of my life. On his desk were pictures of children that I assumed were his.

"I'll send these out myself, and you give me a call when you want the information. Remember you have to come in for the results."

His voice pulled me out of my momentary reverie. "How long does it take to get the results back?"

"Not long. I won't rush it unless you want me to, so routine time by the beginning of next week."

He opened the door and led me out, the waiting room empty and quiet.

"I'm sorry I kept you late."

"No problem. I stay late a lot. It's a good time to catch up. No interruptions."

I reached out and touched his arm. "Thank you so much for all you've done for me and for Mark."

He smiled. "You are most welcome."

I tried to forget about the testing and the outcome and busied myself with everyday tasks; I taught classes, attended meetings and chauffeured the children back and forth. The teachers at the church nursery school deserved sainthood for taking care of Jake as he leaped, dashed and finally crashed during quiet time. His joie da vivre was in stark contrast to Lucy's time spent there when she had been quiet, diligent and an obedient, busy bee.

Alone in my office one afternoon grading papers, a tentative knock broke my train of thought. Figuring it was a student, I mumbled, 'come in' not looking up.

Sam stuck his head in the door and barked, "Give them all A's and go home. Don't you have kids that need to be somewhere?"

"Well, well," I chided, "look what the cat dragged in. I used to know someone who resembled you, but that was in another life."

Hanging his head, he grinned sheepishly and shuffled into the room. "Yeah, yeah, I know I've been a putz. Go ahead, rail at me and get it out of your system." He grabbed the back of the chair and swung it around, straddling the seat.

Picking up the post-it notes lying on the table, I chucked them at him, hitting him on the head.

"Hey, did anyone ever tell you, you throw like a girl?"

"I hit you didn't I? And if you haven't noticed big boy, I am a girl."

"Yes, you are," he grinned, his eyes slowly taking me in. "And you still have great legs."

For some reason I became flustered, we'd teased about women in short skirts before, but this felt different. I said nothing while Sam continued to watch me in silence. A moment passed.

Wanting something to distract from whatever was happening, I got up from behind the desk to replace a book on the shelf. I felt Sam's eyes following me. Neither of us spoke.

Unused to awkwardness with Sam, I smiled. "It's good to see you. I've missed you."

"Me too."

"We probably should talk."

"I know." He waited a moment before going on, stood up and came over to me. "We'll go get greasy pizza some night soon when you can get a sitter and talk all you want." He draped his arm around my shoulder and gave me a gentle squeeze. "I know I've been out of touch. It's what I do. Actually, it's what I had to do." He let me go and walked to the door. "Pick a night when Loren or someone can do the rug rats and let me know. See you soon."

As I watched him leave, I stood rooted to the spot next to the shelves. It hit me how important he was to me and how I'd missed him being in my life. With his arm around my shoulders holding me close, I felt taken care of, a feeling I hadn't had in a long time.

After the evening rituals of dinner, baths, bedtime stories, and multiple tuck-ins, I fell gratefully into bed thinking how ordinary the days were and how thankful I was for their routine. Life goes on, birthday parties to buy for, cupcakes to make, groceries to pick up, clothes to wash. I thought about Sam, how he made me laugh and this afternoon had made me feel desirable; and always, Lucy and Jake, who gave me a reason to get up in the morning.

I wondered when I'd be able to call Hal for the test results and then, just thinking about it, the dread crept back, stealing in like a peeping Tom, holding me hostage. Rolling over in the bed to the empty space that Mark had left, the tears started to burn, their briny taste lingering on my lips.

How could one human produce so many tears and where did they hang out before they fell? (Remember, this was long before we could ask Alexa.) My head resting in the place where the tears had dampened the pillow, I fell asleep thanking God for giving me the ordinariness of life.

In the dream, I knelt in the white sand on a beach with turquoise water, the gentle lapping of the waves and the cawing of the seagulls, the only sounds. The sand warm and deep, I sunk down, knees buried. My white, gossamer dress buttoned down the front and my hair, loose, fell over my shoulders, blowing slightly in the cool breeze from the water.

In the distance I saw a man coming towards me, his footsteps crunching in the sand. Without speaking he dropped down in front of me and reached out his hand to touch my face. Gently, cupping my chin, he leaned over and kissed me, his kiss salty, his lips dry and rough. He stopped, looked me in the eyes and moved his hand gently down my neck, kissing my throat as he undid the first button at the top of the dress. I sighed deeply as he loosed the buttons and kissed my skin in the place where each button came undone. The filmy dress open, he reached both hands underneath the fabric and….

The harsh jangling of the alarm woke me with a start. I opened my eyes and glared at the offending clock face. That was a good dream, one I wanted to finish! Awake now, I sat up, swung my legs over the side of the bed, and burrowed my toes in the thick rug. The sun cast a pale, golden hue over the wet grass, birds were chirping and somewhere a dog barked. I smiled, got up and padded over to the window. The air had changed overnight, officially fall in central Florida. I thought about the dream. *The man of my dreams, maybe life isn't over just yet.* My steps somewhat lighter, I sauntered down the hall into the kitchen to make coffee before the children got up.

That afternoon, I waited in David's office suite comforted by his squishy sofa and listened to the soothing sounds of Windham Hill playing in the background. I loved the way his office worked. You never saw who went in before or after you, appointments were scheduled with exactitude, those leaving, exited by the back door, so only the receptionist and the 'to be seen' patient lingered in the reception area.

The door to his office opened, and I glanced up as David came out. Always struck by his dark good looks, he was a tad shorter than I and even under a jacket, it was obvious that this man was built. Sam, who worked out with him, referred to him as Dr. Huge. He was about Marsha's age, early forties, and tended towards rumpled khakis and non-leather shoes without socks. The tattoo around his ankle spoke of wilder days. In his doctoral student years, he had lived on an island off the Georgia coast, caring for primates. Now he cared for three wild boys, all under ten. A vigilant vegetarian, he scorned all animal products and ate nothing that dreamed. When he shared this last fact with me, I had laughed and asked how he knew which animals dreamed. All of them did, he declared.

"Hi, you're looking almost rested." He ushered me in the open door to his private office.

"Thanks. I slept last night. No Xanax. No nothing. Just one kick ass, good dream."

"Well, with that opening you know I'll need details."

"Yes," I murmured and lowered myself into the usual chair, not making eye contact with David.

"Well, you just went from up to down and I don't mean the chair. What just went on there?"

"For a fleeting minute I forgot the real reason I come here." I lifted my eyes not saying anything. Silence hung in the room. With an audible sigh, I told him about getting tested and waiting to find out.

"Wow. That took guts, you know. When do you think you'll feel like you can hear the results?"

"I don't know." I eyes trailed over the diploma filled wall. "I really don't know."

"That's okay," David nodded. "You were brave to do it and now it's done. You wait until you are ready. It may be days, or next month, but you've made the decision that you knew you'd have to make eventually."

I thumbed my fingers on the chair arm. "It's like I've taken a leap off that treacherous ledge and now I may hit bottom or I may catch myself on a limb, like that recurring dream, like I'm on some journey, stuck in some horrible place and if I can ever get wherever it is I'm going, I'll survive."

"And to get there you had to take that leap off the ledge. Like you have."

"I know."

"Now, your dream, the one that made you feel so light," he smiled.

"My dream, was glorious." I grinned. "It felt so real and intense that I could swear the man in my dream was in the room caressing me."

"Sounds like a keeper. Who was he?"

"Don't know. He just arrived in the dream, knelt in front of me and unbuttoned my clothing, then kissed me gently when each button was loosened. I woke up as he pulled me toward him."

"So in the dream you felt…."

"Oh, I felt loved, cherished, beautiful, free, light. When I woke up, I was smiling."

"Stay with that feeling for a minute. What's going on with your body right now? Your face?"

I rolled my eyes toward the ceiling, dismissive.

"Humor me."

"Okay, but it feels silly. Here goes. My eyes are light, sort of like butterfly wings, not heavy and teary like they have been for so long. My mouth…" I pressed my lips together and then opened my mouth and ran my tongue over the top lip. "My mouth is like not shuttered up, not needing to hold back the lump that has been in my throat for so long."

"So how does it feel?"

"Feel?"

"Yeah, how is it not to feel buttoned in?" He waited. "The buttons in the dream and the undoing them."

"I never thought of my feelings as being buttoned in."

"Maybe not, but sometimes when I watch you it seems difficult for you to let things come out. We've talked before about you being so comfortable in your head and how you tend to have trouble with your heart."

I didn't respond immediately but sat still, my hand covering my mouth.

"What's your hand doing now?"

"Huh?"

"Your hand. It's covering your mouth. Kind of like holding it in. Buttoned."

"I always do that. Sometimes I sit in meetings and get so irritated with what's going on that the only way I can keep silent is to literally cover my mouth."

"What would happen if you let whatever out?"

"Dear God, I might say the awful things that I'm thinking."

"Why is that so bad?"

"I don't know. Sometimes I'm so un… uncharitable." I paused. "Maybe I'm afraid."

"Afraid of what?"

"What I may say. It may hurt someone. Cause pain." I waited and a frown worked around my mouth. "And," my eyes fell, "let others know my weak spots. Make me vulnerable."

"Vulnerable, huh, how would that be?" David leaned forward in his chair.

"I, uh, I don't know. Not good. Scared."

"Scared of what?"

"Yesterday," I began. "Yesterday, Sam came to see me."

David nodded.

"And he apologized for being gone for so long. He was, well, you know him, he was Sam. He told me I had great legs, but it felt kind of different from the usual Sam comment. I was flustered, embarrassed almost."

"And what did you do when he complimented you?"

"I retreated. I guess I 'buttoned' up. I didn't know how to respond." I focused on the wall.

"How would it have felt to say thanks for the compliment?"

I forced my eyes back to David, "I don't know. I didn't realize I didn't say thanks." I paused. "I guess it would have been okay."

Suddenly the jangling noise of the telephone pierced the quiet in the room. No one called during sessions unless it was an emergency.

"Sorry." David slowly rose from his chair and crossed the room to his desk. He picked up the phone, listened, then said it was Marsha for me.

I got up and walked slowly to the phone.

"Marsh," I hesitated. "What is it? Are the kids okay?"

"Oh, thank goodness." I sighed with relief. "I'm to call Dr. Jacobsen?" My voice rose. "Did he say anything?"

The only sound in the room was the barely audible strains of Windham Hill playing in the background as I stood fixed, listening to Marsha on the other end of the phone.

"No, I'm okay. I'll call him. I have the number. No it's really all right. David is here. I will. Thanks. Bye." I hung up the phone and turned to David.

"Hal called my office, said he needed to talk to me." I rubbed my hand around the base of my neck and drew in a deep breath.

Focused on the telephone, I raised the receiver and cautiously punched in the phone number. Out of the corner of my eye I saw David going quietly to the door.

I mouthed in a stage whisper. "Please stay."

He turned, nodded and lowered himself into the chair across from where I stood.

The phone in my hand, I eased down at David's desk. One elbow on the desk, my head propped in my unsteady hand, I gripped the phone and closed my eyes wondering what had gone wrong with the test? Would I have to do it all over again? Had someone found out? I just prayed. Minutes passed, the only sound in the room the monotonous clicking of the clock.

My eyelids fluttered open as Hal's voice came on the line.

"Hello, Hal. Yes, no, I'm in David's office. Yes, he's here too." My eyebrows rose, my voice puzzled, "What? You have the test results. But you said I'd have to come in."

David edged forward in the chair, his gaze fixed on me.

"Oh my God," my voice broke. "Are you sure?" Tears filled my eyes and raced down my cheeks, my shoulders shuddered.

"No, I'm all right. David's right here. Yes, I know, I know," I stumbled. "Hal, thank you so much. I'll let David know." I laid my head down on David's desk and sobbed, my body shaking.

David bolted from his seat and crossed the room in two paces. At the desk, he bent over and touched my arm.

"I'm okay," I whispered and lifted my tear stained face.

"I'm so glad. That's what I'd hoped." His eyes crinkled, filling.

I smiled through the blur of tears. "I'm really okay. I tested negative. That's why he called."

David moved around the desk and put his arm around me hugging me tightly.

"I can't believe it. I'm really all right." Letting go of David, I pulled a tissue from the box on the desk, wiped my eyes, blew my nose and fell back in the chair.

"That means the kids are completely fine. They're healthy." I breathed deeply, "And we're safe."

"You are." David leaned back on the edge of the desk looking down at me.

Hearing him, it hit me that a portion of the malignant fear I'd lived with was gone for now. I needed to pinch myself to make sure it wasn't a dream. After all these months of being so afraid and now I'm not infected and even more, the kids can't have it.

David smiled at me.

"I know that I'll probably have to get tested again, but I'll never have to worry about the children, never again."

"No, you won't. You should be tested again, but you waited almost a year, so this test is as accurate as possible at this point."

I let the tears spill into the edges of my mouth. I liked the way they tasted. "It's over for now."

"Yes, it is. You took the leap and survived." He waited and then continued, "What now?"

"Huh?"

"What do you want to do right now?"

"Right now," I stopped. "Right now, I want to tell Marsha and Annie. And Sam, and call all my Boston folks. And then go home and hold my kids." My face grew solemn and my voice quiet. "And Mark. I need to call Mark. He'll be relieved to hear we are all right."

"I imagine he will be."

"It will make it different now, knowing."

"How?"

I didn't know, I just knew it would be.

Chapter 10

Like an ultra-light on its maiden voyage, I glided from David's office down the sidewalk, taking in the familiar sights as if seeing it all for the first time. Even the usually seedy storefronts in the small town, appeared fresh; the shop windows with their bountiful Thanksgiving cornucopias overflowing with red and yellow Indian corn, the gaily colored mums spilling out of flower baskets; not unlike a New England Thanksgiving season, just a perfect 80 degrees and no sign of early snow. This place needed an ice cream shop, heavenly Haagen Das. I'd order the largest dulce de leche they had, and savor the sweet, cold custard as it melted and dripped down my chin.

Glancing at my watch, I realized I could just catch Marsha and speeded up the pace. On the steps to Marsha's office, I bumped into Sam, who was on his way out.

I beamed at him and told him I wanted to find Marsh before she left for the day and that running into him was an added bonus.

"Well, glad to be a bonus. What's up?" he set his satchel down and leaned against the wall.

I gushed with the news, "We're all okay!"

He grabbed me, lifted me off my feet and spun me around. Putting me down, he opened his arms to the sky and yelled out at the empty street, "Dios es bueno. God is good!"

I began laughing and crying at the same time as Marsha stepped out the door.

"I heard all this racket." Turning to Sam, she chuckled.

He bowed at the waist. "I've just been given amazing news that demanded a proclamation."

"So I heard. God is good. Is it what I think it is?"

I told her the news and she reached out, tears rushing her eyes and hugged me close.

Not to be left out, Sam grabbed both of us in a fierce grip, kissing us one after the other. "Shall we go celebrate?"

"I can't today. I've got to go pick up the children," I grinned at him.

"And I've got to go to the store, so I can pretend to make dinner for the family who lives in my house," Marsha added.

"All right, I can see that I'm out voted cause of familial obligations. We'll celebrate later, though."

"We will. I've got to run." I paused. "Thanks for being my friends no matter what."

"We love you!" Marsha shouted.

"Me too."

That evening, I was energized, on fire, as the kids and I grilled hot dogs and toasted marshmallows. Lucy was picking hers off the coat hanger and licking sticky fingers while Jake purposely let his catch fire.

"Eeww, gross, Mom look at Jake's. It's all black."

"I like it that way. I eat fire," he bellowed and opened his mouth wide, cramming the charred marshmallow in.

"Mommy," Lucy said. "I want hot dogs and marshmallows every night. It makes you happy."

"Honey, you and Jake make me happy. And I do love hot dogs and marshmallows too, but I especially love you." I leaned over and kissed Lucy.

"And daddy too," added Lucy, looking directly at me.

I avoided Lucy's eyes. "Gosh, it's late. School tomorrow, time for bed, guys."

After stories and tuck-ins, I sat down at the kitchen table staring at the phone and considered the day. Wow! *Thank you Lord, I murmured a silent prayer, you must not be ready for me yet.* I needed to call Mark and call my parents about Thanksgiving. We were going there for the holiday. Mark, on the road with the rock group, said, he wouldn't be coming. With the testing behind me for now, it was time to talk to my folks. Sharing the whole sordid mess would be difficult and their reaction to Mark, difficult to gage. He had been like the son they never had.

My mother answered on the first ring. We chatted about arrangements, and I told her Mark was traveling so he wouldn't be joining us.

"Well, I'm sorry about Mark, honey. We wanted to see him. But, he must be doing okay, since he's traveling and all."

"Yes, he seems to be doing all right." I hesitated. "I'm going to run. I need to call Mark before it gets too late."

I hung up the telephone and dialed our house hoping Mark was home. It turned out he was in Boston for a few days between shows. The group was making headlines, their tapes were everywhere, and they had a European tour coming up this spring. We chatted for a bit and then, I shared my news.

Mark's voice broke. "Thank God. It's what I hoped for. I thought you were, but now I know for sure." Relief evident, he continued, "And the kids, the kids were always all right. It was you I was worried about."

"I know." I waited. "Me too, but I don't have the virus. I'll have to be tested again, but I went for so long that the test is as accurate as it can be."

Mark breathed deeply into the phone, husky with tears, "I love you and it'll be okay now. We can go on. You don't have it."

I wavered, uncertain of how to continue. "So, I'm taking the kids to my folks for Thanksgiving. We'll leave next Wednesday. Are you going to the Cape?"

"No, I don't know what I'll do. I think everyone will be at my brother's, and I'm not sure I'm up for the chaos."

"I get it," I laughed. I'd always needed a break after the hubbub of holidays with the extended family. "Well, we'll be in Jacksonville gorging on southern food. Listen, I've got to go, it's late and I need to call Annie to tell her the good news. At some point, now that we know the kids are okay, you probably need to tell the rest of your family the truth."

"Yeah. Probably."

"So, we won't see you until when?"

"I don't know. Soon. We need to talk about the move and what you're bringing."

"We do," I replied, my voice steady.

"You'll be here after classes end, I figure."

"Let's discuss it later."

"What do you mean, discuss it later?"

"Just what I said. I want to talk about it some more when I see you."

"It is already discussed. You and the kids are coming home before Christmas. To stay."

"Mark," I demanded. "I don't want to talk about this now. I need to go. Good bye." Exhaling, I hung up the phone and leaned against the wall fearful that Mark would call back. Seconds passed and the phone did not ring. Relieved, I dialed Annie's and shared my news.

"Thank the Lord. I am so relieved, not that I didn't know it already. I knew God wouldn't let me lose you. It's that faith thing I have going on."

"I know, Annie. I wanted to believe it too, but reason got in the way."

"Honey, it's that head of yours. You need to spend more time listening to your heart."

"Hey, you been talking to my shrink?"

"Well, you could just pay me. You know I'm good." Annie inhaled as she spoke.

I smiled thinking of Annie, propped up by her phone, the fan blowing overhead as she sneaked a late night cigarette, the door to the porch open.

"Are you smoking?"

"Of course, I cannot tell a lie. Gary (her boyfriend) is dead to the world. My ciggies are my second vice."

"Second? What's the first?"

"Good sex."

"What?" I whined into the phone. "Did y'all just do it or something?"

"A quickie in the bathroom."

"That is more than I need to know," I laughed.

"Well, it's the reason I'm up smoking this late. A smoke after sex is just the best. Those old movies had it right. I keep hoping I look like Lauren Bacall in her slinky nightgown if I hold the cigarette just right." She paused and took a drag. "I am so glad you are okay. I knew you would be, you know."

"You did say that. And it is cause you love me but now it's true. I'm exhausted and going to bed. I'll call you tomorrow. Night."

"Night, honey. Sweet dreams."

The following week, the children and I drove north to Jacksonville for Thanksgiving. Traveling through the state forest, dense with old growth pine and majestic water oaks, their branches provided a shelter over the winding road. Spanish moss was draped like a crocheted shawl over the protective arms of the trees, and I was struck by the natural beauty of a place I'd seen many times, only now, really seeing it. Once again, I breathed in and prayed thank you. The windows down in the station wagon, I inhaled the cool wet air, relishing the quiet. Jake had fallen asleep about halfway, and Lucy busied herself with headphones and Care Bear tapes.

Soon, I pulled into the fifties neighborhood where I grew up. The confederate jasmine, still fragrant, wound around the wrought iron posts on the front porch and the ancient camellias stood sentinel awash with pink and white blossoms held up by waxy green leaves.

As the car stopped, Jake woke up, rubbing sleepy eyes.

Lucy bounded out of the car and up the front steps to be first to ring the doorbell. Not to be outdone, Jake, now fully awake, slipped the confines of his seat belt and vaulted to the porch stopping momentarily to snag a low hanging camellia.

The door opened and my dad leaned down and scooped Lucy up in a bear hug. Jake dashed past Dad, brandishing his prize camellia and he and Lu ran toward the kitchen shrieking for Memaw.

I opened the back of the wagon and took out our bags.

My dad leaned over, gave me a kiss and told me to go on in.

"I'll get this. Of course, your mother has been worried." He raised his eyebrows and grinned.

"And, of course, when is she not?" I laughed back. Going up the steps, I paused, surveying my dad's handiwork. All his tender plants had been moved to the porch and many were still blooming. Frost could come to north Florida by about Christmas, if not before, and Daddy would fret about losing plants. Every year that I could remember, I helped him lay sheets over the flowering shrubs and tender perennials. Every year he would bemoan the loss of a favorite and vow not to plant it again, which he always ignored. I hoped it would never change.

That night after the children were in bed, I nursed a cup of tea in front of the crackling fire. The temperature had dropped to the forties and true to southern traditions my mother had lit a fire. Daddy sat in his favorite chair and stoked his one allowed pipe of the day.

"Tom, I do wish you wouldn't smoke that old thing. It just smells up the room and you'll end up with throat cancer," my mother chided.

Not pausing in his pursuit of pulling on the pipe, Daddy shrugged as he cut his eyes to me. "Sounds familiar, huh?"

"Well, honey you know I'm right. It will give him throat or mouth cancer and it does smell."

Taking the pipe from his lips, Daddy responded. "It's been smelling for about 40 years, and I don't have cancer yet. We all have to die with something."

"And Mom he's down to one pipe a day. That's quite an improvement."

"Well, yes. It's just that I'm sort of fond of the old coot and I'd like him to stay around."

Dad smiled at her and continued to puff.

We sat in comfortable silence for a few moments, the only sound the popping of the fire.

It was time. "I need to tell you something."

Attentive, Dad put down the maligned pipe.

"And, Mother," I directed. "I need you to not get hysterical with this. Just listen and don't say anything until I finish."

She frowned at me. "Whatever you say, but I don't always get hysterical, you know."

I took in a deep breath. "Mark doesn't just have cancer. He's HIV positive. He has the virus that causes AIDS, and it will eventually kill him."

My parents stared at me. I quickly raced on.

"The children and I don't have it. I just got tested last week, and I know I'm okay and the only way they could have it is through me, at birth."

"Dahlin, where did he get it?" my dad asked, deadpan.

"He's not sure, but he had sex with someone who must have had it."

Mom's hand went to her mouth, and she let out a weak gasp, "Oh, my Lord."

Dad rose from his chair and moved to the sofa next to Mom. He patted her knee gently. In a manner of fact tone, he asked, "Who did he get it from?"

"He hasn't said. I'm not sure he knows."

My mom burst out with, "What? He doesn't know!"

"Yes."

"But he got it from having sex with someone?"

"I thought AIDS was a homosexual disease."

"Well, no, not really. It can affect straight people too."

"So, did Mark get it from a man?"

"I don't know, Mom. Like I told you he hasn't said."

"So what about the cancer, does he have cancer?" Dad asked.

"Yes, Daddy it is cancer, but it turned out that the cancer was a result of the HIV. I couldn't tell you before now because I didn't know about me and the kids. I couldn't tell you until I knew we weren't infected."

"Good Lord, child," Dad leaned forward. "We're your parents. You've been dealing with this all alone, and we should've known, we could have helped."

My eyes teared up. "I didn't know how to tell you that we might be dying. I was so scared."

My mother got up from the sofa and put her arms around me. "Oh, honey, whatever you did or didn't do, it's all right. All we care about is that you and those precious babies are healthy. I just thank the Lord that y'all are okay."

"Dahing, your mother's right. I just can't bear to think that you went through all this alone." He turned to my mother. "It all makes more sense now. I told you something wasn't right. Just never would have figured this." He shook his head. "Your mother had such trouble with you not being up north with Mark. It made no sense to her."

"Your mother! We both did, you know that Tom." She went back to the sofa and plopped down beside him.

"Yes, yes, we both did. But now, my Lord, it's a good thing Mark isn't anywhere near here." He scowled, got up, and knocked his pipe out into the fire. "I can't believe the man I've cared for like a son all these years has behaved like this. Risking you all's lives. What the heck was he thinking?"

"Kathy, honey, who else knows about this? Mark's family?" Mom asked.

"No, just Phil, his brother, who has been really helpful through it all with the medical stuff. I don't know when Mark will tell Jack and the rest."

"Well. It's clear that you're not going back to Boston now."

"No Dad, I'm not. I haven't told Mark yet. I have told him we need to discuss it, but he doesn't want to hear it."

"Well, he'll listen when you don't go."

"Are you going to divorce him, honey?"

"No, Mom, there's really no reason to. I'd lose out financially if I did. I think he'll pitch a fit when I tell him we're staying in Florida but then get over it. I actually don't think he cares much about anything I do. He just wants to be with the kids."

"Makes sense, dahlin." My dad's voice was tinged with sadness. "I'm real angry at him, but you know, I'm also sorry for him. He's lost it all. What a waste."

Chapter 11

Thanksgiving Day dawned cool and overcast. Mom cooked turkey with all the trimmings for our small family and the neighbors next door. The children eager to finish dinner, gulped turkey and dressing and were playing outside when we heard Lucy's excited screech, "Daddy!"

I glanced over at my dad, excused myself from the table and hurried to the front door. Through the top transom I saw Mark kneeling with Lucy in one arm, Jake tucked under the other. It took a moment to collect myself and I walked quietly back to the dining room letting them all know Mark was here.

Mom looked up, said nothing for a moment, then her southern hostess manners kicked in. "Well, imagine that! Tom, did you hear that, Mark is here. Go tell him to come on in."

"No, Dad stay in your chair. I'll go get him."

Turning to their guests, my mom continued, "We didn't think he'd get away, with how busy he's gotten lately."

"Well, we're just so glad he's getting better. What a horrible scare that cancer was for you all."

Dad avoided their eyes and busied himself by carefully cutting his piece of pecan pie. He said nothing and took an extended swig of the iced tea.

I returned to the dining room with Mark. His eyes surveyed the table smiling at Mom. He bent down and gave her a quick kiss.

"Come have a seat, and I'll get you some dinner," she offered and started to rise.

Mark touched her shoulder, "No, I've eaten already, please sit down." Looking up, he greeted Dad and the guests.

Dad did not get up immediately but waited and cut his eyes to Mark. A knowing moment passed between the two men and then, recovering his inbred good manners, he stood and grabbed Mark's hand, holding him in a half hug.

"Good to see you. You're looking well."

"Well, thanks. I'm feeling a lot better. It's just good to be here with my family," Mark smiled and looked at me.

Suddenly, the front door slammed and the children came running into the house, their excited voices filling the quiet. Lucy reached the dining room first, Jake close on her heels, both children going on about a huge turtle in the yard.

"A turtle that big, huh. This, I've got to see. If you all will excuse me." Mark nodded to the table and was dragged out of the room by Lucy.

I sat back down and fiddled with my pie. As dessert finished, Daddy got up and led the guests into the den. Mom began to clear the table.

I told her to go sit and let me do clean up. It would give me something to do.

"Well, all right but I think you should be outside with Mark. Is he all right with the children?" she asked, her voice anxious.

I was surprised and puzzled by my mother's concern. She'd been a nurse. "Of course he's all right. He's perfectly fine with the kids. Why wouldn't he be?"

"Well," Mom fretted with a corner of the tatted place mat, holding it in front of her like a shield. "He's got AIDS. And honey, we don't know that much about it."

"Oh, Mom," I reached out and held her close. Having lived with the diagnosis for so long, I hadn't thought about the fears that my parents might have about the contagion of the disease. "He's not contagious. You only get it through sex, and needles. If it was easy to get, I'd be dying."

"I know, I know, it's just that I worry so about the children, honey. If anything ever happened to them and to you, it'd kill me." Her eyes filled.

"Mom, we are fine. We really are. I promise."

"Ladies," Dad's voice boomed into the dining room as he stuck his head in. "We have company, did y'all forget?"

Dabbing her eyes on the corner of a napkin, Mom whispered, "He only can entertain for so long and then he wants to go sit and read." She grinned over at him, "No, I'm coming. Kathy is cleaning up."

The evening passed quickly. Mark did baths and tucked in the children. He came back into the den and sat in front of the fire.

Conversation was stilted and avoided any mention of what I had shared.

"Well," Dad yawned. "I'm beat. Gonna call it a night. What about you?" He asked Mom as he got up and walked to the door.

"Well, I'm a little tired myself. Good night, y'all."

Mark and I sat in silence across from each other staring at the fire. Finally, I brought up the move to Boston.

"You heard me." I repeated firmly, "I said, I'm not coming to Boston."

"I heard you all right. I just don't believe what I heard."

"Mark, I'm not moving. I'm not living with you. We're staying in Florida for now." My voice rose.

Mark stamped over to the fireplace, his back to me, his hands gripping the mantle. He said nothing for a moment as he stared down into the fire.

"You'd really do this to me," he muttered and slowly turned around to face me. "You'd keep me from my children when I'm dying just to pay me back."

"I'm not keeping you from your children. You can see your children whenever you want. You travel all the time and you can come and go from Florida as well as Boston, you know that."

Mark glared at me and in one fluid movement, crossed to where I sat, grabbed my arm, and jerked me to my feet. He grasped my shoulders with his hands and began to shake me.

"Stop it!"

He shoved me and losing my balance, I tumbled backwards over the arm of the sofa banging my back on its edge as I toppled down.

Lying there, I heard my dad's enraged voice, "Just what in hell do you think you're doing, Mark? Good God man, have you lost your mind?" He dropped beside me on the sofa and cradled me in his arms.

I'd heard my dad 'cuss' maybe three times in my life. He always said cursing was for folks who had poor vocabularies. I stared up at him.

Mark remained motionless, frowning down at us.

"Are you okay, honey?" Daddy gently put his hand on my cheek.

I touched my back where it had hit the hard armrest. "I'm all right."

"She stumbled and fell," Mark commented, his voice even.

Ignoring Mark, I carefully lifted myself from the sofa.

My father stood up, his fists clinched by his sides. He faced Mark. "I have known you like a son, and I have loved you like a son. It is utterly beyond my comprehension that you could have done this to your family, but you have." He shook his head, "I just thank the good Lord, that they don't have it." He raised his hand and pointed his finger at Mark. "If you ever, ever touch my daughter again, you will be dealing with me and trust me, you don't want that." Whirling around, his back to Mark, he shot back over his shoulder, "And I imagine you'll be leaving in the morning."

I woke up to the memory filled aroma of perked coffee, threw on the robe that lived on the closet door hook and went into the kitchen where my Mother was busy making pancakes. Daddy was outside fussing with his plants. I didn't see Mark. Giving mom a good morning kiss, I poured a cup of the thick, black syrup-like coffee into the large mug set out on the counter.

"Morning honey, I know you need something to lighten up your daddy's coffee. I swanee you could stand a spoon up in it. There's cream in the refrigerator, real half and half. I know it's bad for me, but it's one of those things I just can't let go of." Mom paused, her hand on the spatula, and told me Mark left real early.

"Your daddy told me what happened." She turned off the stove. "Let me look at that bruise."

"It's fine, Mom. I fell and just hit my back."

"I can't believe that man! Shoving you like that in this house. I nevah!"

The back door slammed as Daddy came in. "I was right ungentlemanly with Mark." He took a mug from the cabinet and filled it with coffee, black. "I had coffee with him this morning and suggested he leave before you got up."

I'd seen my dad really mad one other time, like he seemed now, when he threw the Jehovah Witness folks off my grandmother's porch. The anger was palpable and so unlike him.

Trying to ease some of the pain, I added, "You know, Mark's not okay, I mean emotionally too. I know that. But he loves his kids."

"Well, I'm not sure he knows the first thing about love, dahling," Dad added sadly as he took Mom's hand.

Chapter 12

On the drive home I replayed the scene with Mark over and over, his fury, the pushing. It was frightening.

Lucy was subdued and wanted to know when Daddy would be home. In all honesty, I didn't know, but assured her it would be soon. She seemed to be satisfied with that and busied herself with her newest tape. I got the children unpacked and settled in for the upcoming week of school, work, and what had become their routine. I'd just taken a long bath and was ready for bed when the phone rang. It was Sam. I filled him in on Thanksgiving, leaving out the shoving incident. I don't know why.

"Mark being there must have been nice for the kids. Maybe not so nice for you, but ..."

"Actually, it was awful. We fought. My dad asked him to leave and Mom cried." I paused, "The only thing good was the food. I ate too much."

He said nothing for a moment then, "Damn, Kath, I'm sorry. You don't need any more to deal with. Listen, what about I take you to supper tomorrow night. No kids just us. See if Loren is up to staying with them."

It all worked out and the next night at the local Italian place, facing uninspired pizza and cold beer, I sat across from Sam in a back booth picking at the pizza, not eating much.

"You should eat," Sam prodded. "As one of three kids, I never turn up my nose at free food, no matter how bad it is."

"You really do eat anything. It's probably why you rave about my cooking. And don't give me that poor kid, no food crap. Your folks have plenty for God's sake."

"Yeah, but my dad works all the time."

"And they own a damn ranch in south Florida!" I laughed. I knew I should eat, I'd get sloshed if I just drank. "Cut me another slice, please."

Sam smiled and sliced through the gooey cheese with the pie server, handing me the oozing steamy piece of pizza. "And if you get sloshed, I could take advantage of you."

Frowning at him, I took a large bite and then a quick gulp of beer burning my mouth. "It's hot," I yelped, fanning my mouth.

"Duh, when steam is rising it usually is."

"Stop. You told me to eat."

"So, drink up and chow down babe. It'll do you good. You need to let go once and a while."

"Could it be that you and Dr. Huge have been talking about me?"

"Not today we didn't." He shot me a slow grin, "You know him, tight lipped, shrink type. We do talk about your legs, though, chauvinist pigs that we are."

Smiling, I swigged the cold beer, then put down the mug and stared at Sam, silent for a moment. I wanted to talk to him about the night Mark told him, but wasn't sure how to start and not sure I should go there, but the new 'get out of your head' me wanted more. So, I just jumped in. "I only just realized what you told Mark that night, the night he told you the truth and you were so angry."

Sam looked at me and said nothing.

Uncertain of how to continue, I ran my index finger around the rim of the frosted beer mug and waited, not my strongest talent. I couldn't stand the silence anymore, so I blurted, "You said that you, that, you loved me." I gazed down into the mug and went on before I chickened out. "Actually, I believe your words were something like, 'God dammit, how could you have done this to your family' and you pointed at me like I wasn't really there. And then, you stared at me and said 'I love her and I love your children.' Then, you got up and looked daggers at Mark, swinging the beer bottle." I raised my eyes to Sam. "Do you remember all that?"

"Wow." He shook his head. "Quite a memory." His voice turned serious. "I remember it all. I remember how I felt after it happened. I wasn't fit for people for a while so I took off. I told you, it's what I do." Taking a swig from his beer, he put the mug down and rubbed his forehead, shoving back his hair. "You remember all the details. I didn't think you were even there, emotionally. I mean I saw you, I knew you were there physically, because you came in to the middle of it."

His eyes traveled over to the plastic grapes gathering dust, hung from the netting on the wall, "I know you had just showered and had on a white gown, your hair was down and still wet. I was so aware of you and then not at all. Mark was my friend, you were his wife." Hesitating, he went on, still avoiding my eyes, "It was usually the way I felt around you."

I didn't know what to say. Neither of us spoke.

I finally broke the silence. "So what you said, what did you really mean?"

"I said I loved you, I'm just not sure how. You're Mark's wife." He raised the beer mug and peered over the glass, "Those words have always gotten me in trouble." He grinned, "Love, not wife. More beer?"

I shook my head, uncertain of what to say.

"What do you want to do now?" he asked.

I paused, not answering and looked straight at him. "I don't know." I knew I wanted to be with him but after that I wasn't sure. "What do you want?"

"Let's get out of here, grab a few cold beers and go somewhere special. C'mon." He reached over and helped me out of the booth.

In the parking lot we climbed into his Jeep and pulled slowly out into the street. He stopped at a 7 Eleven to get beer. Back in the car, he handed me a cold Coke.

"Thought you might not want any more beer, just yet."

"Thought you were gonna take advantage of me."

"Baby, if that happens, I want you to remember it."

We drove in silence, the cool breeze fanning my face as I leaned back, eyes closed. The car came to a stop in the parking lot by Sam's office at the college. Not sure of what we were doing, I held back.

"Trust me." He took my hand and led me down the alleyway to the back of the building. The alley ended in a small fenced backyard, lush with vegetation. He took out a key and fitted it into the heavy gate. It swung open.

The pale, yellow glow from the waning moon cast a gilded light over the shadowy outlines of low hanging fruit trees. I could feel Sam's breath warm on my neck, his hand on my waist, as he guided me over the uneven path, the heady fragrance of the ripening fruit laden on the trees, almost overwhelming. The moon shadows danced on the damp grass, reflecting the abundance of tropical flowers lining the lush borders of the garden. Awestruck, I had no idea this place existed.

Moonlight lit the way as Sam took my hand and we stepped onto a patio with lounge chairs, side table and a long wooden garden bench. Alive with the night sounds of crickets and peepers, the outdoor symphony was punctuated by the occasional screech of a heron as it swooped over the treetops. Speechless, I lowered myself to the bench and gazed up at the brilliant night sky.

"The heaven tree of stars hung with humid nightblue fruit." Sam's voice pierced the silence.

I gazed over at him as he stood silhouetted by the moonlight realizing this young man never ceased to amaze me.

"Say that again, it's beautiful."

"James Joyce, Ulysses. The heaven tree of stars hung with humid nightblue fruit."

He sat down on the bench beside me.

My face close to his, I was scared. Not really scared, like frightened scared, just sort of scared like I don't know what to do, scared.

He put his arm around me and drew me close as I leaned my head on his shoulder. Gently he put his hand under my chin and kissed me softly on the mouth. He stopped and stared at me. This was the moment when I knew that I would take the leap off the edge, go with my heart, and ignore my head which was screaming logical thoughts like, *are you crazy, this man is about 14 years younger than you, you are married, your husband is dying, you have children, oh my god, what is the matter with you?* So, I leaned toward him and returned his kiss. Cautiously, he kissed the cleft in my neck and unbuttoned the top button on my shirt. I sat motionless, hardly daring to breathe as he kissed the space where the button was undone. He asked me if it was all right. I mumbled.

Slowly, focused, he undid each button and kissed me in the space where the button had been fastened, like in my dream. The shirt undone, his fingers lightly brushed my breasts.

I gasped, my breath ragged.

He raised his eyes and looked carefully at me.

In a whisper, I told him about my dream. "It was you. You did this in my dream. The way you undid the buttons and then kissed me and then the dream was over. And Sam," I gushed on, "I haven't been with anyone but Mark since we were married. I'm not sure what to do next, and, but I do, and I'm scared and I'm not...."

He put his finger to my lips, stood up and lifted me off the seat, guiding me to the lounge chair. "I want to make love to you more than anything, but I need to know if it's all right for you."

As scared as I was, I knew. "Yes, I want you to." I drew in a deep breath.

Taking his time, Sam held me with his eyes.

"Kath, look at me. It's just me here with you."

Breathless, I let go, the tears filling my eyes. A few moment passed and I sat up in the lounge chair.

Sam perched on the end of the seat. He reached over and laid his hand on my leg. "You okay?"

In the dim light, I smiled. "I'm fine."

"I realize that this is huge for you." He traced his finger down my jaw. "And for me."

"I'm really okay. It's you I'm concerned about. You know you're young and all that."

Sam burst out laughing, "Right, my beautiful older woman. Like Mrs. Robinson you have taken advantage of this impressionable young man."

"I didn't mean it that way. I just..."

He gently covered my mouth with his hand and shifted closer in the lounge chair. "Don't speak. Just be." He took his hand away and kissed my mouth.

Minutes passed while we sat in comfortable silence and listened to the night sounds; crickets, peepers and car horns somewhere in the distance.

Getting up, Sam disappeared into the blackness beyond the patio. I could see him, white, outlined in the backlight of the moon as he reached up to a tree in the yard. Bearing a large grapefruit in one hand, he kissed me and sat down on the bench.

Moving in the half- light I sat down next to him while he efficiently removed the peel, stacking the peeling on the table by the bench. Inserting both thumbs into the moist fleshy fruit he broke the grapefruit apart and held a piece out to me. I nodded and he put the sweet, tart fruit between my lips, the juice dripping down my chin. With his wet thumb he wiped my chin and traced a line to my lips. I took his thumb in my mouth savoring the sweet, acid taste of him. Taking his hand down, he tore the grapefruit into sections, laying it carefully on the table.

Silently, I watched him sitting there, naked, but for his opened shirt, his elbows on his knees crouched over the low table, a handsome man, so physically different from Mark. I loved the way his hair curled on his arms and the strength, yet gentleness, in his hands. He's so young, I thought, and yet, not so young. I must really be over the edge. I've just made love with a man in his twenties, my husband is dying of AIDS, and I'm savoring the taste of grapefruit like I've never tasted it and loving the sticky juice as it runs down my chin.

"You've been quiet for at least 2 minutes. Are you breathing?" Sam teased.

"I was just thinking."

"That's too bad. Gets us in trouble."

"No really, be serious." I paused, "You're quite a risk taker. This is a lot."

He didn't say anything for a minute and looked intently at me. "I am a risk taker. That's true. I also give blood as often as I can so I know I'm healthy. I know you are okay. That's the physical risk piece for me. The emotional risk," he paused, "well, that's an unknown. I know I won't lose our friendship. The intimacy makes me feel closer to you. It adds intimacy to an already close friendship. What could be better than that?"

I smiled at him.

"And, mi amore, it is a lot. But life is a lot and it's what we are given and what we have now, and the beer is still cold, the nightblue fruit sweet, the moon is full and you," he cupped my chin in his hand, "are a beautiful, bright woman who is not dying, and we are here with each other under this 'heaven tree of stars'. What more could we ask for?"

Chapter 13

The time between Thanksgiving and Christmas flew past. The semester ended and infused with gratitude and the Santa Claus spirit, I baked cookies, wrapped toys and sang along to the familiar carols. Sam was with his family, and Mark was coming Christmas Day to take the children to Disney through New Year's. I'd arranged to go to my parents and would be home by week's end, when Sam and I planned to have some time alone. We'd been together with the children, which was not unusual, but hadn't been alone for any length of time since the night in the garden. I'd fretted every which way about that, not sure how unhinged I really was and what it all meant, and then, finally just given it all up to the universe. Both Marsha and Annie provided much needed solace and humor, pruriently demanding all the details. I smiled and treasured that night's intimacy, sharing little.

Lucy and Jake hung up their stockings on Christmas Eve and as I tucked Lucy in she asked why daddy wasn't with us. With solemn eyes and a hurt expression, she snuggled into me.

"Oh honey," I pulled her close. "Daddy would be here if he could. He's working. He'll be here tomorrow"

"Don't you love Daddy anymore?" Lucy scooted away from me.

I said nothing for a moment. Then, I reached out and put my hand on Lucy's shoulder.

"Your daddy and I are apart, but we still love you and Jake very much. I know it's hard for you and that you miss him. I miss the way it was too, but we can't live together now. So we have to do it this way."

"But do you still love him?"

I sighed and looked away. *How do I this?*

Lucy put her small hand out and grasped mine, gazing up at me.

"It's okay, Mommie. He loves you. I still love Daddy. And you too."

I stared at my earnest, young daughter hoping to get this right. "My dearest angel, we love you more than anything and that will never change."

"Will you always love me?"

"Of course."

"But if you stopped loving daddy, you could stop loving me too."

I grabbed Lucy into my arms and clutched her tightly.

"Baby, it's not like that. Grown up's sometimes stop loving each other, but when you have a child you never stop loving them. You are a part of me. You lived inside of me for almost a whole year and I loved you then. And then you were born and I've never once, not loved you. I love you more than anything in the whole world."

Lucy looked up and a slight smile lit up her small face.

"More than anything?" She grinned, crinkling her nose. "More than duckie de lucky ice cream?"

"More than dulche de leche ice cream and more than," *all* my shoes!"

Lucy laughed and threw her head back, shaking her hair back and forth, "You are a silly billy, mommie."

"And you are a sleepy, snuggly, sugarplum who needs to get under the covers so Santa can come."

"That rhymes, Mommie," Lucy giggled and burrowed under the light down comforter. "Cover me up to my chinny, chin, chin and don't let the bedbugs in."

Smiling down, I kissed her on the head, nestled her in the covers and turned off the light in the bedroom.

"Santa will be here in the morning if I go to sleep real fast. And Daddy too. Night Mommie."

"Yes, my darling baby girl, they will both come. I love you. Good night."

I went in to the kitchen and got down my Christmas present from Sam. I'd coveted the almost translucent wine glasses and before he left he'd surprised me with six. The previous year, (before the world shifted) on my birthday, he and another colleague had given me a good bottle of Chardonnay, and I'd assumed that the other man had chosen it. He was older, after all. Sam bristled at my misplaced appreciation and reminded me he was young, not ignorant. How far I'd come in understanding that! Pouring a glass of the Cabernet I'd opened earlier, I swirled the wine around, admiring the way the glycerin coated the balloon glass. Taking the wine to the living room, I plopped down on the sofa and slowly sipped, savoring the earthy plum taste and the peaceful solitude.

The twinkling lights on the Christmas tree played off the glass ornaments, the paper chains Jake made dressed the mantle, and Lucy's clothes pin reindeer added childlike simplicity to the nativity. I suddenly felt overwhelmed by an enormous feeling of loss, coupled with immense gratitude. The familiar tears welled up and I let them come, coursing down my cheeks embracing their salty brine at the corners of my mouth. With the back of my hand, I swiped them away and took a sip of wine. Soon, the glass was empty.

I glanced at the clock and realized that as the single Santa Claus I needed to get busy. Quietly padding down the hall, I carried unwrapped big presents from the closet to the tree and arranged them in piles, one for Jake and one for Lucy. Hidden in the kitchen cabinets were goodies for the stockings. I filled each with fruit, candy and small toys, pausing at Mark's stocking which Lucy had hung up next to hers. Gathering more candy and fruit from the kitchen, I filled Mark's stocking. Presents were under the tree for Mark, so it only made sense that Santa wouldn't forget Daddy.

After putting the presents out and filling the stockings, I stood back and appraised my handiwork. Not too bad for a single Santa; a bit different than a year ago, which seemed a world away. With a sad smile, I turned out the lights on the tree.

Muffled noises entered my consciousness and I cracked open one eye as Jake's small hands pulled at me. "Santa's been here and Daddy's here too!" He burst out of the room and darted down the hall.

My arm covering my face, I lay still. So, Mark had come in time for Christmas morning. He must have gotten the red eye special and driven in the wee hours. His energy level was incredible. How he could keep up the pace with his illness amazed me. Then again, all our friends always said he was the one who would steal the spoon and dig the tunnel to get everyone out of the prison camp.

Stretching my arms over my head, I listened to the excited sounds of the children from the living room where Santa had been. Sleep still lingered and uncertainty made me wary about how the day would go. It was Christmas, I was Pollyanna (as Mark had said, and he was partly right) so I was eternally hopeful, but Thanksgiving had been miserable. I sat up on the side of the bed, my feet touching the floor and slowly stood. In the bathroom I washed my face and rinsed out my mouth. Uneasy, I fiddled with the snarled hair around my face encouraging it into some semblance of order, slipped on my robe and padded down the hall into the Christmas melee.

Mark looked up as I came into the living room. His handsome face drawn, circles under his eyes, he looked exhausted and even thinner than he had at Thanksgiving.

"Merry Christmas," he said.

"Merry Christmas," my voice catching, I tried not to gape at his emaciated appearance.

"There's coffee in the carafe." He held my eyes for a moment and looked away.

"Mommy, look what Santa brought me! It's a Teddy Ruskin!" Lucy shrieked, holding up the talking teddy bear. "Listen to all the things he can say and he sings too, listen." She pulled the ring on the teddy's back and his sing song voice began.

Jake sat mesmerized on the floor, already constructing a large pirate ship with his newest Legos. He barely looked up as Teddy Ruskin began to sing.

I smiled, glad Santa had done so well and went to get coffee.

Soon, the room was knee deep with paper, boxes and trimmings. One small box wrapped in telltale turquoise paper and tied simply with a silver ribbon remained under the tree.

Jake spied it, picked it up and announced, "This is the last present. Is it for me?"

Mark laughed, the lines around his eyes deeply crinkling in his gaunt face. "No buddy, that one's for your mom. Santa left her something."

Jake reached over and handed me the simply wrapped package. I stared at Mark and said nothing.

Both kids eagerly bounced around offering to help me open this surprise gift. Grinning at them, I slipped off the ribbon and tore open the paper. Inside was the signature Tiffany's box holding the turquoise jewelry bag.

"Ooh, look at that little bag. Can I have the bag Mommy? It will be a good purse for Teddy." Lucy pleaded.

Mark put his arm around Lucy and hugged her to him, "Baby girl, let Mom open it before you take the bag away."

I opened the drawstring on the bag and reached in, pulling out a pair of classic Tiffany, silver starfish earrings. Taking a deep breath, I looked over at Mark. "They're lovely!"

Mark held up his hand in a 'stop' position. "Glad you like them. I know how you love starfish."

"Can I hold them Mommy?" Jake put out his hand.

I handed the earrings to Jake.

"Put them on, Mommy, they're so beau- tee- ful and sparkly," Lucy sung out. "Daddy got you a wonderful present, huh?" Lucy gazed up at Mark and then stared at me.

"Yes, Daddy did. Thank you, Mark."

"Well, you're welcome, glad you like them," Mark responded evenly, staring at me. "And thank you guys for all my presents too," he addressed Jake and Lucy.

By late afternoon, the presents put away, I got together overnight bags for each child. Mark had napped for a few hours and came into the bedroom as I was packing Jake's clothes.

"You can come with us if you want to. The children would like it you know." He leaned against the doorjamb in Jake's room watching me.

I turned, the wariness returning, Jake's small shirt, a barrier clutched in front of my chest. "I'm going to see Mom and Dad and do some stuff around here."

"You really don't want to be with me, do you?"

"Mark, let's not do this. It's Christmas. It's been a nice day." I looked down and busied myself with the bag. "I'm glad you were here for Santa." I paused, "It's late, if you all are going, you need to get moving."

He regarded me coldly. "I just need to understand one thing. Why are you doing this to us? This family. You know it doesn't have to be this way." He came over to the bed and sat down heavily on the edge looking up at me.

"Don't start this, please."

Reaching out, he pulled me down next to him on the bed and leaned into my face, his breath medicinal and sour. "I will not let you take my family away from me. Do you understand that? Nothing is going to stop me from being with my kids."

I jerked my arm away, got up and crossed the room to the doorway. "You just don't get it! And you don't want to get it. I have never intended to take your 'family' away. You took it all away when your behavior risked our lives. And now," enraged, I vented, "now you want it all to just go away, and for us to go on, like it was a happy family. Only, only, there's one small problem. Daddy's got AIDS and Mommy thinks she's okay and well, the kids, the kids, that Daddy LOVES SO MUCH aren't infected because, because of God's grace and good karma."

Spent, I exhaled, my voice now quiet, "You know, Mark, I pray every night for God to take care of you and to give me the strength to forgive you. I don't want you to die without me learning forgiveness."

Seething, Mark stood up without speaking and brushed past me in the doorway.

I stood there, shaking, waiting in the silent room, the sick smell of him lingering.

Chapter 14

It was late afternoon when I pulled into the carport and began unloading the car after a peaceful visit with my folks. Not having the children at my parents' house was strange at first, but we soon established a quiet routine; reading by the fire, walking to the water, good wine and uninterrupted dinner.

My empty house felt cold and hushed, kind of lifeless. I guess I was already missing the kids. I looked around, shuddered slightly and turned up the thermostat. Wood sat stacked in the bin by the fireplace and in minutes, I had a crackling fire. I poured a glass of thick Syrah (it was winter, after all), put on Vivaldi and settled down on the sofa. As I watched the fire my thoughts rambled: what were the children doing now; I should call my folks to let them know I was home safe; and I hadn't heard from Sam.

A loud banging at the door startled me out of my reverie. Still for a moment, I wondered whether to pay attention or ignore it. The noise continued, so I got up and parted the sheer curtain, peeping out the window by the door.

Sam stood with his head resting on the door. "Hey, I know you're home, I checked out the car. Let me in or I'll huff and puff!"

Laughing, I opened the door, and he burst in, swung me around, and then held me back at arm's length telling me I was just beautiful.

Loving to hear such flattery, I tilted my head back and grinned, asking him if he was drunk.

"Only, mostly drunk." He pulled me toward him and kissed me hard on the mouth.

"Sam, you ARE drunk, I've never seen you drunk."

"Well, I'm just only, mostly drunk," he whispered, took my hand and kissed my palm, gazing up into my eyes. "Now if we were in Princess Bride, I'd have you right now, my pretty."

"Come in and have some coffee before you have me." Taking his hand, I dragged him into the kitchen, "Sit. I'll put on the coffee."

"I'm not really drunk, just a few plane drinks and no food. Food would help." He glanced around, asking about the kids.

I told him they were at Disney with Mark and there was food in a minute. Not waiting he went to the refrigerator as my eyes followed him. Faded jeans and a sandy v-neck sweater wrapped his muscular body like loose packaging. Loafers, not flip flops graced his feet. I started to sweat, thinking about the night in the garden. "Aren't you back early?"

"Yep," he answered, and removed the Tupperware dishes from the refrigerator, setting them on the counter. "God, this stuff looks great," he lifted a lid and poked his finger in the dish.

I swatted at his hand. "You're worse than the kids! I'll get a fork."

"Taste this. It's amazing." He dug his finger into the mixture and put it up to my mouth.

Now sweat was glistening on my brow. Holding his eyes I took the food off his finger. Not speaking, he took another finger full of casserole, putting it to my lips. Just like that, I let him feed me, savoring the sweet taste of squash like I'd never tasted it before.

He ran his hand from my mouth to my throat and slowly slid down my neck. At the first button on my shirt, he stopped and grinned.

"Sam, I...".

He laid two fingers across my lips, then took his hand down, slowly undoing each button until my corduroy shirt was hanging open.

I stood paralyzed, not speaking.

He parted my shirt and bent down. "Now what were you saying?" he glanced up under his eyelids.

Gasping, I leaned against the counter for support.

He slowly reached up, his hand around the back of my head and undid the clip that held my hair. It cascaded down, falling over my shoulders. He moved away and stared at me.

I smiled.

We lay on the rug and watched the fire burn down, covered by the sofa afghan, the only sounds in the room the settling of the ashes and our breathing.

"So, how drunk were you, really?" I asked, trailing my finger along his jawline.

"Not very. Not enough to get in the way." He kissed my finger.

"So what brought you back early?"

"The extended family in New York is great but really, boredom and you brought me back quicker."

"Me?"

"Uh huh. You."

"It's nice to have you here. I'm glad you were bored."

"Me too. Are you hungry? Cause I'm starved. What's in all those dishes?"

"My mother's specialties that she makes at Christmas. Most of it is obscenely bad for you but wonderful."

He got up and pulled me to my feet.

I smiled at him. "Let me get some clothes on."

"Why? Are you cold?"

"No, I'm just not sure about eating, naked."

"Well, it's a perfectly fine way to eat. Clothing just gets dirty." He leaned in and kissed me. "You seem good. Rested and calmer. Things are better?" he questioned.

"I am, better and calmer. It was really good to go home. I missed the kids, but it was nice too, to just be with my folks." I paused, "Things with Mark are no better. The more I stand my ground about not going back, the more he pushes."

"Well, he wants you all with him. I can't blame him for that." He waited, "And Mark is not someone who takes no lightly."

"I know. That's what concerns me."

For the first time in months, I slept deeply, no dreams. Sam had stayed the night, and I woke with his arm resting on my belly. It should have felt awkward, sleeping in a bed with another man after all my years with Mark, but somehow, having Sam there seemed comfortable. It was no longer our bed. Mark hadn't slept there in almost a year! And maybe, my sheet burning ritual did have magical powers. Carefully, I slipped out from under the caress, not wanting to wake him.

One eye flickered open as he reached out and pulled me back close to him.

"I didn't want to wake you up."

"I'm always half awake. I gotta be ready," he mumbled, nuzzling my hair.

"Ready, ready for what?" I laughed and tried to wriggle out of his arms.

In one fluid motion, he flipped me on my back and pinned me down, my arms in a tight grip over my head.

"I can't move," I whined and grinned up at him.

"And?"

Holding both my arms with one hand, he leaned over, kissed my neck and continued down my body teasing me with his tongue until I cried out.

"Stop," I moaned, half laughing. "I can't take it anymore."

"You give?" he asked, peering up at me and released my arms.

I grabbed for him pulling him up to my face.

Afterwards we lay sweaty and spent, the covers in a tangled heap beside the bed.

"Thank you for making love with me," Sam said softly and kissed my forehead.

"I loved making love with you. It's like dying and then not."

"You know that the ancient religions felt it was as close as you could get to the Divine or the Mother."

"Well," I touched his face with her palm. "They had some kind of insight, didn't they?"

"That they did, but it threatened the hell out of the mainline power mongers so here we are, sexually repressed and tearing up Mother Earth."

We lay silent, my head resting on Sam's chest. Moments passed with only the quiet ticking of the clock breaking the sounds of our steady breathing.

Finally with a long sigh, Sam got up from the bed, slipped on his jeans and sweater and coming back to the bed, gave me a light kiss. He needed to get home since he'd come to my house directly from the airport. I smiled, and told him I'd planned to stay in bed for a little while longer.

"Go back to sleep. It's not often that you get to sleep in. I'll let myself out."

I was still, my head propped up on the pillow realizing that the leap right off that huge cliff of vulnerable was really all right. I was all right. Inhaling, I pulled up the covers, which smelled like Sam, a lingering aroma of lemon, soap and earth. I closed my eyes and must have drifted in and out of a light sleep, because I woke slowly to the sound of the front door opening. Sitting up, I

A Red Door

swung my legs over the side of the bed. Sam must have forgotten something. I walked to the closet, slipped on my robe and went down the hall.

"What'd you forget?" my voice sang out. In the doorway to the kitchen, I stopped abruptly.

Mark stood by the coffee machine and stared at me. His face was drawn and ashy with deep circles under his eyes.

"Mark! What are you doing here? Where are the kids?"

"You were expecting someone else?" Mark responded in a monotone, his eyes taking in my robe and disheveled hair.

My voice shaky, I gestured towards the front door asking about the kids and why they were back early, was someone sick?

"The children are fine. Asleep in the car." He turned away, reaching into the cabinet for a cup. "Want a cup?" he asked, his back to me.

"Sure." I went to the refrigerator, got out the cream, and put it on the counter. He poured coffee into a cup for me as I stirred in the cream and pulled out a stool next to the kitchen bar. The only sound in the kitchen was the whirring of the refrigerator.

He put his cup down and sat on the other kitchen stool beside me. "It appears that you were expecting someone else?" He bent his face close to mine.

I inched back, stared directly at him and waited.

"Now, I understand why you won't come home."

"It's not why I'm not coming," I glared at him, "home, as you put it. And what I choose to do is none of your business."

His mouth curled up and his voice rose, "It is my business. You are still my wife. And you have my kids. I won't have them with you and some lover you've taken up with."

I shot up and frowned down at him. "How dare you throw morality at me! You, of all people. I am your wife on paper only and apparently have been that way for a long time. And as for our kids, this has nothing to do with them."

Mark stood, his face in mine. "And where is he now? Out buying the Times? Flowers? Oh," he tapped his hand on his forehead, "of course, you must have used all the condoms?"

My hand flew out, but before it connected with his cheek, he grabbed my wrist and pulled me toward him.

"You never were that quick, my dear. Physical prowess isn't your strong suit."

"Let me go." As I twisted to free my arm, the loosely fastened belt on my robe came undone.

With my arm gripped in one hand, Mark lightly brushed the swell of my exposed breast with the other. "Why are you afraid of me?"

"Mark, I mean it. Let me go," I raised my voice and tried to keep my robe together with my free hand.

The phone on the wall rang.

Mark dropped my arm, "I'm sure you don't want me to get it."

I moved quickly and reached for the jangling telephone.

"Hey, it's me. Don't let on, just pretend that it's Annie or someone," Sam spoke, not giving me a chance to say anything.

"Hi, yes, I'm fine."

"Well, I know that's not true. I left my sunglasses there and was coming back by when I saw the rental car in the driveway and one small head lolled over in the car seat. I figured it was Jake in the seat, and that Lucy was inside with you."

"Mark got home early with the kids. They're still sleeping, but Mark and I were just having coffee."

"He's right there."

"Yes."

"I'm down the road at the 7-11 at the pay phone. I decided to play it safe and call. Also, wanted to be sure you were all right. Should I come by?"

"No," I looked to Mark. "I'll catch up later. I think Mark is leaving soon."

"Are you sure?"

"Yes. That's fine with me."

"Okay, I'll come by when the car is gone. God, I'm sorry about all of this."

"Yes." My back to Mark, I hung up the phone and faced the wall taking in a deep breath before turning to face him.

Just then, the front door banged open, and Lucy flew in, running to me and circling me around the waist.

"Mommy, mommy, we had such a fun time with Daddy! You should have been there and seen me ride the huge-est space ride ever, and Jake threw up in the body ride but I never did," Lucy exclaimed, barely pausing to take a breath.

"Sweetie, I'm so glad you all had such a grand time." I squatted down to hug her. "I missed you so much."

Lucy giggled and wriggled out of my arms. Taking my hand, she smiled over at Mark, "Daddy, let's show Mommy what we got in the car." She pulled me to the door. "She's gonna be surprised, huh?"

I cut my eyes to Mark. He said nothing.

As we approached the car I could see Jake beginning to wake up. He stretched in the car seat and rubbed his eyes with clenched fists. When he saw me, he grinned. "Mommy, mommy, come get me out."

I reached into the car and freed him from the seat. He clung to me and nuzzled his face in my hair. "You smell like my Mommy."

I kissed his damp forehead. "And you smell like my sleepy headed boy."

Holding Jake, I went around to the back of the car as Mark opened the trunk. In the trunk were two riding toys, a small blue bicycle and a Big Wheel.

"See, Mommy, look what else Daddy got us!" Lucy jumped up and down. "Take it out for me to practice, take it out Daddy, pleeeease."

I stared at Mark as he began unloading the toys. "Well, these are great. Christmas comes twice."

"Yes," Mark nodded. "They seem pleased. They can learn to ride them here and bring them to Boston when they come home. By the way, my family knows the whole story and is ready to help out. So, there's one less hurdle."

Puzzled about the family news, I held my tongue. His mom had mid stage Parkinson's and it was all his dad could do to care for her. I was on the phone with Phil, his doctor brother, at least a couple of times a week, and he'd shared with no one. The other brother who lived near us on the south shore was busy with five kids, and I wasn't sure he'd been told the truth because I was close to his wife and she probably would have called. His sister in Maine was a bit removed but still kept up. The cousin/sister was tight with Mark so I expected she had been told, but if there was a side to take she'd be with Mark. Perhaps, Mark had only told his dad and if so, I'd speak to him soon.

Chapter 15

To my relief, Mark left late that afternoon. He said nothing more about the move and appeared to engage himself with small household tasks. That night I called his folks to wish them Merry Christmas and thank them for the money for the kids' presents. His mom's voice was weak and unsteady as she passed the phone to Jack, his dad. The first thing out of his mouth was a monologue of sorrow and pain and worry for me and the children. It was probably the most emotionally wrought conversation I had ever had with the man. I assured him we were fine, and that I was sorry to have to do it this way, but it was all I could manage at this point. He ended with an 'I love you' which I'd never heard, and then shared with me that he felt closer to me than he did with his daughter. Dumbstruck, I cried and his voice broke. We'd talk more later, we both promised.

The next few, post- holiday days were comfortably filled with lazy mornings, bike riding practice and easy suppers, sometimes including Sam. School and work started back mid- week, and I had an appointment with David.

Nestled in the familiar chair, I was lulled by the quiet gurgle of David's new meditation fountain. When I closed my eyes, I had a sudden memory of Mark's hand skimming my breast. An involuntary shudder traveled through my body. How could I feel so uncomfortable by the mere touch of someone I'd loved?

David's voice brought me back. "You seemed so relaxed a moment ago and then you just gave a serious full body shudder. What's that about?"

I opened my eyes and glanced over at him telling him about Mark's visit and the impact it had on me. I guess I was so happy spending time with the kids and had a nice holiday that I kind of forgot about it until I sat down here.

"You have good coping skills. Putting unpleasant things away is an effective defense mechanism. It allows you to go on in spite of bad things happening. We just move them aside from our conscious thoughts and then wham, they hit us the face at unsuspecting moments." He paused, "Want to talk about it?"

"Not really, but you'll make me anyhow."

"Well," he grinned, "I'll encourage you strongly."

I didn't say anything for a moment and then related the scene in the kitchen where Mark held my wrist and touched my breast. When I finished, I noticed my hands trembling.

"He means to scare you. It's his way to control. You need to limit the times you are with him and not be with him alone."

"David, he won't really hurt me. It's just intimidation." I stopped. "He looks terrible. He's all grey and smells like medicine. He's dying."

"He is dying, but he can be dangerous, dangerous to you and to the kids."

"Oh, David, he loves the kids. He would never," I hesitated and looked directly at him, "never willingly hurt the children. I know this much."

"Then why do you seem afraid of him?"

My eyes filled, and I looked away.

David reached over, took the box of tissues from his desk and handed them to me. The gurgling of the small fountain filled the silent room.

"You know how we talk about you being in your head and how that kind of response is comfortable for you." He waited, then continued, "The fear response you have about Mark is the opposite. It's "gut" stuff. It's a protection device."

Keeping his eyes on me, he sat forward in his chair. "Listen to it."

Blowing my nose, I wadded up the tissue, and clutched it in my hand. "Do you think he would really hurt me?"

"I don't think so, but I know what Mark did to your family. Clinically, some narcissism seems like it takes over." He shrugged. "I think he's unpredictable. And I think you need to get legal."

"Legal?"

"Legal. Call an attorney and find out about legal separation, custody, child support. All the things that you need to know about."

"But, David. He's dying. I don't need to do all that stuff."

"I think you do. I think he may not die for a while. Mark is a young, strong man and has access to the best medical care. He will do all he can to get what he wants."

David fixed me with a hard stare before continuing, "And he will stop at nothing."

I kept my eyes on David for a moment and then gazed away. "You know, I thought that I loved Mark so much and that whole time, I honestly believed him when he said he didn't know how he got AIDS."

Shaking my head, I went on, "I felt like such an idiot, so stupid, when he finally told me the truth. Then those months of not knowing if the kids and I had it, I was always waiting to slip down into the pit and just holding on to the edge, barely. And then, then when I knew we were okay," I rubbed my naked ring finger, "it was like I had another chance at living." My eyes shifted back to David, "I slept with Sam."

I waited for him to respond, expecting some comment. He said nothing.

"It was like nothing I ever had with Mark. With Mark, it was hot, fast and passionate and then, in the last year, almost nothing. When I think back, it had gotten pretty routine and impersonal even before that. We had great sex, but I'm not sure we made love a lot."

I hesitated. I'd never said anything about this to anyone. "Mark washed his hands."

"Washed his hands?" David raised his eyebrows.

"Yeah," uncomfortable, dropping my eyes I fiddled with the shredding tissue. "After we had sex, he'd go into the bathroom and wash his hands."

"How did that make you feel?"

"I didn't like it. It was weird."

"And you felt?

I swallowed. "Like I wasn't clean."

"Did you ever say anything to him about it?"

"I think I asked him once."

"And what did he say?"

"I don't think he really said anything."

"And with Sam you said it was nothing like with Mark. What did you mean by that?"

"Well, with Sam it was slow, lingering and so intense, so intense that I lost myself."

I continued, relishing the memory, "Sam was so there. So totally there. No one else existed in the whole world but Sam and me. It's been like that every time with him."

"It sounds like making love with Sam is good for you."

"Good for me! I lose all conscious thought." I grinned at David. "I think I see stars and might die."

David smiled back. "I think that's what folks write and sing about." He paused, "I think also that you trust Sam and allow yourself to let go."

"I never felt like that when I made love with Mark."

"Well, maybe, you never really trusted Mark."

"David, I had children with Mark. What do you mean?"

"I wonder if your unconscious knew something, that your conscious mind didn't, something that remained there hidden and it kept you, like a protection device, from completely letting go with Mark."

"Why? What was it protecting me from?"

"Well, maybe if you had really let go, totally trusted, you might have pushed more on the sex thing with him."

I froze, saying nothing.

He waited. "You didn't."

"You mean, maybe some part of me knew."

"Not really knew, but kept distant. Kept safe in some way. Our defenses work for a reason. Sometimes they are primitive, but right on."

Chewing on my bottom lip, I tucked a stray hair behind my ear. "So with Sam, I trust him and let go completely because my gut tells me it's safe."

"In a way, yes."

"I may really love Sam," I frowned, the idea unsettling.

"That's not a bad thing," David shook his head. "Sam's a good man."

"David," I shot back. "He's 26 years old and I just turned 39."

"And?"

"Well, he has his whole life to live. I have kids," I reasoned. "I'll be 40 soon."

"Forty isn't exactly an end of life moment," he chuckled. "Some of us do manage to move about and take nourishment. And believe me, you won't get in Sam's way while he lives his life. He's a pretty independent and able guy."

I got up and walked to the window, my back to the room standing there for a moment. "Falling in love with Sam isn't what I should be doing right now."

"No one can control when they fall in love," David smiled. "I think it was Voltaire who said, 'to reason about love is to lose all reason.' By now you must know that we have little control over anything. We're given the deck and how the cards play is out of our hands."

As I drove back from David's office, my thoughts were more confused than when I'd gone in. I couldn't imagine how I might be falling in love with Sam; it seemed like one of my craziest fantasies, dream- like, really. This whole affair was probably a transition phase, because even the idea that I could be in love with Sam was insane. He made me feel amazing, alive, desirable, things I desperately needed to feel. Love couldn't figure into this. And certainly, not for him either. Good Lord, he was much younger, had his life to live and I had young children.

And, let's not forget, I had a husband, a husband who was dying of AIDS. Although, the 'terrors' had receded from my daily thoughts, the fears of HIV infection were still with me. Articles appeared in the paper or I heard news stories of someone who had tested negative in the past and now years later had the disease. I knew I'd need to be tested again, and then I could put it to rest, but going through the test again was such an emotional hurdle, and anticipating the test another piece of the fear. Before, the test had been the lesser of the two evils; I was living as though I would die. Now I was living and grateful. I'd only been with Sam, and from what we knew, it was difficult for a woman to infect a man, and Sam tested himself repeatedly as a blood donor.

So the only real test was time and living with fear over time was ultimately debilitating. Sort of like an invisible scarlet letter, the A for AIDS. It would affect any relationship I might have, though I couldn't imagine being with another man at this point.

Mark's cold animosity was chilling. He was certainly in tremendous physical and emotional pain, but ironically, it seemed he was now the wronged party. His anger at me for leaving him ran deep. Egocentrism, narcissism, whatever the clinical phrase didn't matter. David was probably right. I needed to get legal advice, much as I hated involving lawyers.

I pulled the car into the driveway, got out and was putting my key in the lock when I heard a loud wolf whistle. Turning, I saw Sam strolling up the drive.

His voice carried, "You are all I was wishing for, a long, cool drink of a woman." He quickened his pace and reached my side, a wide grin splitting his face as his eyes traveled down my body.

"And you are a brash and audacious flirt."

He wrapped his hand in my loose tee shirt and pulled me to him, kissing me deeply.

I drew in a sharp breath and fell against the wall of the front stoop. My keys and purse tumbled to the floor. "We should probably go inside."

He nodded.

I picked up the purse and keys and fumbled with the lock as we stumbled into the door.

"The kids are at friends," I mumbled and Sam hurriedly pulled my shirt over my head. "They'll be home soon."

"Then we'll have to hurry."

Suddenly, the sounds of laughter and small voices came down the driveway.

"Well, damn!" I fled, shirt in hand into the hall bathroom, just as Jake bounded into the door.

When I came out of the bathroom I heard Jake giggling and begging for 'mercy'. Sam had Jake on the floor and was tickling him as he cried out laughing.

"Hey, buddy," I smiled down at him.

Laughing, Sam got up, shook himself off and pulled Jake to his feet. "Well, that was a different kind of exercise than I had in mind," his eyes meeting mine.

"I know what you mean," I grinned back.

Jake tore off down the hall and I flopped down on the sofa.

Sitting next to me, Sam took my hand and gently brushed his lips to my palm, "You think we could finish what we started, maybe tonight?"

"Nothing I'd like better. I'll see if Loren is around."

"Call her now," he insisted.

"Yes sir."

Coming back into the room, I told him she would be here at 6:00.

He chastely kissed my cheek. "See you then."

I was giving Loren last minute instructions when Sam came in. Jake and Lucy were again mesmerized by the Mary Poppins' video that Mark's dad had sent for Christmas. I reminded them about bedtime when the movie was over, kissed them both good bye.

I asked Sam where we were going as I climbed into the Jeep.

He responded by placing his hand on my leg where my khaki shorts ended, playing his fingers under the edge.

"Soon," he answered.

We rode in silence, the warm wind blowing my hair out of the clasp.

Sam reached over, punched play on the tape deck and the heartfelt sound of Joe Cocker filled the car with the strains of his plaintive lyrics. We drove west for a while into the setting sun.

I studied Sam, sunglasses perched on his straight nose, his face bathed in the watermelon hue of the fading light. His dark hair curled around the back of his neck and his arms glistened in the damp evening air. He gripped the steering wheel with his left hand and his right remained resting on my thigh. I closed my eyes, put my head back on the seat and felt the tension of the day begin to ebb away.

As the car bumped off the tarmac, I opened my eyes to an orange grove. We bounced down a dirt road through the trees and came to a stop in front of a small lake. The sun shimmered on the horizon and washed the languid water with a persimmon glow. Getting out of the car we walked a short way into the grove. As far as I could see, the trees laid out a linear pattern which seemed to reach all the way to where the earth met the sky. Laden with ripe oranges, the heavy branches rested on the rich dirt, the fragrant aroma in the air thickly sweet, the humming of the bees the only sound.

It was amazing how the groves were laid out, Sam told me. Seems it's all a matrix and if you know how to go you don't get lost; perhaps, a good metaphor for a life. I'd never been in a grove before, not this in and I just thought they were planted in rows like other orchards. Hand in hand we strolled out of the grove as the full moon began its rise over the lake, the light, ultraviolet, illuminating our way back to the car.

Sam flipped back the seat in the Jeep, revealing a cooler and blanket. We put the blanket down facing the lake as the moon cast its pale winter light on the black water. Opening the cooler, Sam got out two beers and Vietnam era insect repellent. In companionable silence, we nursed our beers until Sam reached over, taking my hand, and let out a deep sigh.

His eyes studied my face for a moment and then he looked away, speaking into the dark, "You know, when I said that I loved you, that night in front of Mark."

"Yes."

"Well," he turned back to face me, "I do."

"You love me."

"I'm in love with you." He paused, "It's the damnedest thing. I knew it that night when I said it to Mark, but I didn't really know it." Stopping to take a sip of beer, he continued, "Know what I mean? You're Mark's wife, the mother of his children, and I'm a young schmuck who doesn't need to screw up your life more than it is already."

I sat, not daring to move, the only indication that I heard was the throbbing pulse in my neck.

Sam glanced at the water and edged towards me on the blanket.

All I could think about was my time with David today, and my admission that I was falling in love with Sam. At first, I looked at the affair as my need for validation, that I was desirable and worthy. He was about fourteen years younger and had a whole life in front of him. I had so much stuff to deal with and it wasn't over with Mark. He was so angry with me for leaving him and would take that out on anyone I was with. I didn't want Sam to have to be involved with that.

I spoke. "I know that you will leave me."

Sam began to interrupt and I put my hand to his mouth. "No, let me finish." I went on, "You won't leave me to hurt me. You'll leave because other things will come up, other opportunities, options, people." I raised one eyebrow and regarded him carefully. "Other women, too. I'm years older than you."

Reaching over to me, he leaned forward and with his index finger gently traced my jaw line. "Kath, other women have ceased to exist for me since you." He moved closer, and kissed me softly on the lips. "I don't have any answers to all this, but I can't, not do it. I've tried. I've told myself a thousand times to get out. And I did actually. When I disappeared those days after Mark told me, I knew what I'd said. But I came back. I'm in it."

I returned his kiss as we sat under the rising moon, the sweet night blooming jasmine mingled with the heady intoxication of the nightblue fruit as it saturated the cool air.

Chapter 16

I followed through with David's advice and consulted a lawyer, filing for legal separation from Mark, which further infuriated him. Divorce made no sense, because I'd lose out financially and as Mark's wife and widow, I'd be entitled to whatever he had left. We'd always had our own accounts and one joint one which we used for general household stuff. The rent money from the Boston house had gone into that account; the mortgage in Florida came out, etc. Mark had always made more money than I had, particularly when I took time off to be a stay at home Mom, so he kept up with the bills. My salary had covered food, small purchases, utilities and gas. At this point, Mark was consistently paying the bills late, even the nursery program at church and the pre-school teacher that the kids stayed with a few afternoons a week when I needed to be in my office. It guess it was one way he felt he had some control.

Next week was spring break and the children were going back to Disney with Mark. His boy band group had catapulted to the top of the pop music charts and performed at Disney periodically. Nothing could match the incredible attention and opulence provided to the young rock stars, and Lucy and Jake became a part of it when they traveled with Mark. Disney rolled out the red carpet for the entire entourage. The whole pretense that entrapped my kids troubled me, but it proved difficult to out shine teenage rock stars.

Late Friday afternoon, Mark pulled into the driveway behind the wheel of a sporty Miata, electric blue. He had flown in from Los Angeles and though his cough had deepened, his face was tanned and masked the usual gray pallor. Rolling Stone magazine had recently showcased the band and an interview with Mark, a highlight of the article. Jake raced outside to check out the car, while Lucy lingered inside, clinging to her dad.

"And 'on the cover of the Rolling Stone'," Mark flashed me a rare, sincere smile and laid the magazine down on the table. "Thought you might be interested. It's a good interview."

I wanted so much to be happy for him and I was; he'd always needed to be acknowledged, something that was rare in his family. His brother, who was barely a year older had taken all the trophies, real and imagined. Even Mark's graduation from Harvard didn't seem to be enough, nor had his making money by buying land and building a house on Chappaquiddick. I never doubted he was loved, his folks were good people, but damn that Irish reticence and inability to talk about feelings.

He nodded toward the magazine. "We're going to Japan and Europe for the month of May."

"Wow!" I bent over picking up papers and children's books that littered the floor by the sofa.

Lucy watched us both, holding tightly to Mark's hand.

"I want to take Lucy with me."

"I wanna go! I wanna go! Oh Daddy!" Lucy jumped into Mark's arms, nearly knocking him down and flung her arms around his neck.

I raised up and stared at Mark, saying nothing for a moment, just looking at him. When I finally spoke, my voice betrayed me. "Let's discuss this later."

"No. We need to discuss it now. I have to make the reservations, and I've already called the school. They were thrilled. Said what a terrific educational experience it would be."

"She's a bit young for a terrific educational experience."

"I'm not too young!" Lucy snapped back.

"Lucy, go outside and check on Jake. He's been playing in the car for too long. I want to talk to your dad."

Putting her down, Mark patted her on the back. "Go ahead princess, scoot and check on that brother of yours. Mommy and I will work this out."

Lucy looked over her shoulder at her dad and moved slowly to the door reluctantly going outside.

As soon as the door banged shut, I exploded. I couldn't believe he'd done that in front of our daughter.

He shook his head, grimaced and told me not to get hysterical, like I always did.

"Oh, you don't know hysterical, Mark!" I spat back. "You know damn well that if I don't let Lucy go, then I become the bad guy and that she's too young to go half way around the world with a teenage rock group."

"She's not too young to spend time with her father. Lucy is much more mature than you give her credit for. Lucy knows what's going on." He paused to let the next words sink in. "She knows all about you and Sam."

I faced him, speechless.

"You really should be more discreet," he smirked menacingly down at me. "Now that you've made sure we're 'legally separated,' I could file for divorce on the grounds of infidelity."

I was wild. "Get out! Get out of this house right now and do not come back."

"Au contraire, dear wife, this is my house too, remember." Hesitating for a moment, he looked me straight in the eyes. "Be careful. I have nothing to lose in this mess you've made."

Just then the door flung open and Jake ran in shrieking, "Can we go? C'mon, daddy, let's go." He pulled on Mark's hand trying to drag him to the open door, "Mommy, come see Daddy's cool car."

With the children away for the week, Sam and I had planned to go to the Keys. When filled in on Mark's latest salvo, he'd convinced me that staying home wouldn't make anything better. On the trip down we stopped for the night in Ft. Lauderdale to visit a school friend of Sam's. The men fell into their easy, joshing routine as I sat quietly, nursing my beer and pushing bad restaurant food around on the plate. Sam's friend, Michael had recently finished his PhD and taken a job with a local community college, where he'd have time to live, as he put it, in addition to teaching. As I watched the two men I felt old and worn. Neither could remember where he was when Kennedy was shot because he was barely born; Vietnam was a war in history books; and I wasn't sure if Michael, at twenty five, knew that Simon used to sing with Garfunkel.

Back at Michael's after bidding the men goodnight, I fell asleep quickly. In the morning, waking early, I padded into the small kitchen, careful not to disturb the guys and made coffee, taking it out to the tiny terrace. Sitting in the lone lounge chair, I thought back to the evening and wondered if Sam's obvious youth would have been less apparent had I not been exhausted. The age difference hadn't been a big issue so far and last night was the first time it had mattered to me. I'd thought about how the Boston folks, Olivia and Patricia, and the couple friends Mark and I had, would react, because the lens through which I saw Sam usually colored those thoughts. He seemed no different than the other men, just more carefree.

Sounds of waking came from the kitchen. Sam, hair tousled, shirtless, jeans pulled on, coffee in hand walked out to the terrace. Leaning over he brushed his lips lightly on my forehead.

"I couldn't sleep anymore. I was so beat last night that I felt drugged."

"Well, all that crap with Mark has to take its toll." He hesitated, his voice questioning, "You better?"

"Yeah, I guess, I'm better."

"He'll do anything to get to me." I stopped, looking directly at Sam, "And to you."

"Yeah, but I can take him," he teased shoving my legs over and dropping down on the lounge chair. "I'm not afraid of what Mark can do to me. I can handle it all, but I am afraid of what he continually does to you."

He waited for a moment, "When he comes and does what he does, it takes you days to recover."

I started to interrupt.

"No, let me finish. You do really well and almost seem to forget, and then he comes into your life and churns it all up. I hate to see you like this."

He stopped, putting out his hand to lift my down turned chin. "I can only offer some diversion and make you laugh."

I protested that he was more to me than a diversion.

"I know that, but I do those things too. They're good things, laughter and silliness. You will always be fine because you have incredible inner strength, but it's the daily drain of life that gets you down."

"So what do you suggest I do? He needs to see his children."

"He does, but he doesn't need to see you."

"So..."

"So don't be there when he comes and if you are, don't let him engage you. Just hand off the kids and leave if he doesn't."

We left Ft. Lauderdale late morning, negotiating the steady stream of traffic snaking down route 95. South Florida never knew what hit it, I realized, amazed that the fragile peninsula hadn't sunk into the churning Atlantic. Once we passed Homestead, the road narrowed and the first of the Keys' connector bridges began. The water turned turquoise and the vegetation limited to scrub pine and sea grapes.

Checking into an efficiency just south of Key Largo, we unpacked quickly and headed out to the small strip of beach. Sam ran full speed into the water and swam out a good distance until he could no longer touch. I lay down on a towel, relishing the warm sun and the quiet. To be at the beach without pails, shovels, juice boxes and shrieks felt strange, but pleasant, maybe a taste of what life might be when the children were older.

Sam came out of the water and shaking off like a puppy plopped down on the sand beside me.

"I always forget that it's coral out there. Barely escaped getting snagged." He smiled at me. "And I could have seeped vital blood into the water, been chomped by a shark and you'd have never missed me."

Leaning over to him, I kissed him on the shoulder, "You taste salty."

"And you taste," he added, "like night blue fruit." Turning, he kissed me softly on my neck. "Let's go inside"

Lying entwined in Sam's arms, I felt safe. We made love until the light changed and the color outside the window waxed crimson. All thoughts of Mark had vanished like the bright light on the water. Luxuriating in the tender after moments, I closed my eyes and began to drift off. Sam's voice brought me out of my reverie.

"I need to tell you something."

Startled by his tone and seriousness in his voice, I opened my eyes and turned to face him, "What is it?"

"I wanted to tell you before now, but I wanted to be sure about it all."

I wondered if something had happened with work that I didn't know about. Some of the student housing at the college that we'd help start for students with learning differences, (one of the first of its kind, this was prior to the ADA) was in a residential area where it was not welcomed. An expensive lawsuit was in process and no one was sure of the outcome. If the college lost, it would likely move to another location but that hadn't been determined either. The trustees and parents were committed to the future of the school, so 'Pollyanna me' was hopeful something would work out.

Sam continued, "I've been accepted into a program in Jamaica this summer, doing a variety of kinds of village work, building, helping in general, and I may not come back to the college. Maybe start grad school or try to get on with a nonprofit in DC. You know it's been troublesome with the lawsuit and the town and we may not even have jobs. I'll have to see how it goes."

My heart sank and I said nothing, pulling the sheet up to my chin. Of course, he should go, it was a great opportunity, and I knew he wanted to travel and work in something that added to the public good somewhere.

"That's great!"

"It is," he said steadily looking up at me, "but, it takes me far away from here." He stopped, "Far away from you. I applied before all this and us."

"When do you go?"

"At the end of the semester, in May sometime." He waited for a moment, "I'll be gone all summer and may stay longer. I never gave this thing another thought after I applied. I figured it was a shot in the dark, and I wanted to try for it."

My eyes filled.

"I know it doesn't matter when it all happened. But you have to believe me when I tell you that leaving you is the worst of it all."

Once back home, reluctantly, I relented and let Lucy 'engage in educational travel' with Mark for the month. Holding back tears I handed her off to Mark at the airport, then, Jake and I headed for the Magic Kingdom. Jake didn't get why he couldn't go with Lucy and Daddy, but having a special treat with me seemed to curb his disappointment.

Mark was paying this time, so we checked into the hotel, made a beeline for the monorail and entered the make believe world where all "your troubles will be far away." That evening, happily weary, we climbed into bed and Jake quickly fell asleep, still talking about how 'not scared' he had been in the Haunted House, even though he'd squeezed his eyes shut as the ghosts popped out.

Sleep eluded me as I lay awake lost in thought. I wondered what airport Lucy and Mark were currently in; what the month would be like with only one child; and then, finally I allowed myself to think about Sam and the time we'd been together. Although his leaving made me ache, deep down somewhere I knew it was what he had to do. It was inevitable, he needed to live his life, and do what he'd planned to do before we'd begun this 'affair'.

He'd taught me much in this short time, mainly that it was possible to be vulnerable and open to love once again. In some odd way, it had allowed me to forgive myself for leaving Mark, letting me find contentment, and hopefully, in time, to forgive Mark. The relationship with Sam had been ill-fated from the beginning but falling in love was not something you could predict. With these thoughts dancing around, I drifted off to sleep, secure in the realization of how much more whole I'd become by allowing Sam into my life.

In the dream, warm rain blew in gently through the screen, the street lights shimmering on the steamy, slick pavement, the heat rising in a soft haze. I was propped up against the back wall of the porch, my long shirt tickling bare legs, skin hot to the touch, sweat slowly creeping down between my breasts.

We made love standing up, the wall supporting me, the air around us misted with rain. No one else existed in time or space, it was all in that moment. Then, as dreams go, I was alone, on a train, barreling down a dark tunnel. The train rushed noiseless, sound suspended. I held firm as the racing train lurched and buckled, gathering speed. Faster and faster the train accelerated. I squinted, my eyes watering against the pulsing air in my face. Suddenly, the tunnel ended, lights flashed. Vapor rising, the train squealed to a slow stop.

I woke up, startled and reached over to Jake, pulling him close, brushing his sleep smelling, damp forehead with my lips.

The month raced past. At the end of the week Sam would be gone and Lucy would be home in a short while. She'd sent postcards and had a wonderful time with her dad, but I still couldn't help feeling it was all a bit much for six year old.

Though I'd steeled myself against the painful goodbye with Sam, with him facing me, our legs touching under the restaurant table, it was difficult to stay upbeat. The worst thing had happened. We fell in love with each other and here we were. He was going away. And I knew he'd leave me. He needed to go on with his life. I knew it would happen eventually. I just didn't think it'd be so soon.

Sam began to speak.

I held up my hand to stop him. "You're going, and you must. And you need to, and all those sensible, rational statements we've made all along about this relationship." I took a deep breath, realizing that none of what I said meant a damn. I loved him, and was going to miss him terribly. I swallowed, trying to quell the rising lump in my throat, I wasn't going to do this. Any of this. The tears spilled over and ran slowly down my cheeks. "Now see what you made me do," I whined, a vague smile lighting through the tears, as I dabbed my eyes with the napkin.

Sam stared at me not saying anything. The silence lengthened as the soft jazz for lovers wafted from the speakers and the clinking of glasses filled the air in the crowded restaurant.

Silent, I waited.

Finally, he reached across the table and took my hand. "When you're a kid and you play hard and your mom says it's time to leave, you fuss and cry and you hold on and in the end your mom finally pulls you out screaming and you grab your blanket and sob in the car until exhausted, you fall asleep." He stopped and took in a long breath, "Well, that's what I feel like."

I held tightly to his hand.

"You know all the wrong people are in love with each other and the people who are supposed to love each other don't." He shook his head, "It's so damned ironic." His eyes fixed on me, his voice definite, he went on, "Kath, hear me and know that this is true. I don't know a lot. As we've said, I'm just a young schmuck. But know this. You will always be with me and you can never really leave me. I'm a better man with you; I want to know all there is about you; I never get tired of you. It's what they write sonnets about. I just never understood that before you."

Frowning at him through my tears, I squeezed his hand and murmured, "You're not really a schmuck, an ass sometimes, but honestly, I'm afraid I'll never see you again."

"No," he countered shaking his head. "You will see me again. I promise. You'll be somewhere, and I'll be somewhere and one day I'll be where you are."

"But it will never be the same. You once told that if only we could freeze frame life and take out the frames we want to repeat and have it all over again." I waited, "I want to freeze frame us."

"This isn't over for us. I'll be back and I'll write and call just to hear your voice." He sighed, "Just to hear you say 'Hey'. Did you know I love your voice? I love that slight southern lilt and how you pause and then rush fast like you can't wait to say it all. I love your excitement about life. I know that I love you.

I'm not sure what to do with it all, but that doesn't change how I feel. You are the one thing in my life that I know is true." He grinned, "You and my mother."

Looking directly into my tearing eyes he brought my hand to his mouth, carefully kissing each finger. "I love all the fantasizing, thinking of you and always knowing, really knowing how you are for me." He continued, "I am sad, will be sad to not be with you when I'm gone, but my heart and mind are yours. You are the first woman that I've ever really loved. I know that I have it in me to really love someone. All else pales."

"But you really love your mother," I teased.

"Yep, you and my mother. But you may be the last. I'm afraid that I'll always compare anyone else who may come along to you and they will be found wanting."

He'd taught me how to love again and to be whole. What do I do with all that with him gone? I smiled weakly at him, my eyes tearing again. (How could I still have any tears left in there?) I sniffed, and swiped at my eyes.

Chapter 17

With both Lucy and Sam gone, I went through the motions of the day like a woman sleepwalking. I got up, dressed, went to the office to do end of terms tasks, fed Jake, picked up, and anxiously waited for calls from Lucy and mail from Sam. Things at the college weren't looking promising, but we all felt it would work out in the end. When you'd put so much energy, passion and time into a project like starting a college, you had to be a dreamer and a little wacky. The state of Florida was behind us 100% which helped also. Now it was just a wait and see game. Once the federal court ruled, we'd know.

Sometime in the last few days, it had hit me that although I'd been in love with Mark, it wasn't like what I had with Sam. Our relationship had been passionate, intense and demanding, but looking back, something had been missing in it all. I suppose, as David had suggested, I'd never allowed myself that special vulnerability of being entirely emotionally naked with Mark, a part of me always held back. In therapy that one day, David had said it was a protection, a good defense that my unconscious knew something that my conscious mind couldn't handle. That it had protected me.

In mid June, the children were going to Boston to spend the rest of the summer with Mark. He wanted me to come and argued that the house was plenty big for us all. When I declined, he offered to move to our friend's apartment in Cambridge and give me the house. If the college folded, we could sell the Florida property, and the kids and I could live in our old house. He'd be traveling and the Cambridge apartment was available and convenient. I wouldn't need to work, he assured me, as he was making plenty of money. I could be with my New England friends, stay home with the kids and he would not be separated from them. I said we'd see when we knew more about the lawsuit.

Many in the college community ventured away from the stifling Florida summer, but Marsha, as founding president of the college was embroiled in the legal stuff and stayed put. She'd been hounding me to go with her to the spiritualist community, Casadega, about an hour away to have a reading, maybe do something called 'past life regression'. I wasn't sure I even knew what past life regression was but finally agreed. It'd be fun and a nice getaway. Her girls, who sometimes babysat would take care of Jake, so we would have the whole day.

In the car, I turned the air vents toward my face. I wasn't sure I wanted to know what I did in a past life. This one was proving difficult enough to deal with. I lifted my thin shirt up so the cool air could blow on my sticky chest. It was so hot. I moaned. "Anyway, maybe I did awful things and just barely escaped coming back as a roach doomed to melt in the heat."

Marsha laughed as she maneuvered the curvy moss draped back roads. "That's not what this past life stuff is all about. The readers aren't Hindi. We may not find a good past life reader, but I know of a medium who is supposed to be wonderful. She does only positive fortune telling with crystals."

"So, what do crystals have to do with fortune telling?"

"Oh, I don't know, maybe they channel energy or something since they've been in the earth for so long," Marsha replied in her best lecture voice.

"Channel energy, pleeze," I grinned and wiggled my fingers near Marsha's face. "Oooh, come to me great spirits."

"Stop it!" Marsha laughed. "Or I'll crash us and we will be communing too soon with great spirits."

We turned off the main highway onto a bumpy, overgrown state road. No road signs or billboards littered the landscape.

Puzzled by the lack of any development so near Interstate 95 I asked Marsha if she knew where we were going.

"Well, sort of," Marsha glanced over at me. "I've come here before, but I wasn't driving." She gazed straight ahead. "I remember that we turned at the end of this long road and passed a small pond and then it was all eerie."

"Eerie? How so?"

"Well, really quiet and hushed like, no road noises which surprised me cause we're not that far from 95. It seemed like time stood still."

I gave a small shiver and rolled down the window. "Well, time may have stood still, but it's still hot as blazes. They may all have second sight, but they can't control the weather."

Just then, a stiff breeze came up and whipped the trees and road debris. The papers lying on the back seat whooshed by my shoulder as I grabbed for them.

Incredulous, I gaped at Marsha.

"I told you this place was for real. See, it is eerie, just wait till we find the town."

We drove in silence until we came to the end of the road and continued in the direction that Marsha remembered. A mile or so more of the uneven pavement and we arrived on the outskirts of a small hamlet. Bungalows dotted the area around a lake and in spite of the heat, the narrow main street in the town bustled with people walking in and out of shops which advertised mediums, past lives, crystals, hot dogs and palmistry. A shaved ice wagon outside of a large hotel was doing a booming business with a line of customers waiting in the blazing sun. The hotel's wraparound porch was filled with people relaxing in rocking chairs, overhead fans undulating, troubling the humid, hot air.

Marsha pulled into a parking place and we got out of the car taking in the busy town. The town was odd, in a good way. It was hot as Hades outside and folks were out and about and didn't seem to be grumbling. The place should be one more decrepit, dying Florida town and here it was, industrious, like we stepped back in time to when these towns were the lifeblood of farm communities.

"I *told* you and you doubted. It is a special place, settled by spiritualists in the early 1900's to have a place of their own, probably to avoid persecution by the mainstream religious zealots around here. No advertising, no directions, just a lower case place on the map." Marsha offered.

We stepped into a shop for cold drinks, and Marsha shared that she'd called ahead to make appointments for both of us. "I think she just sees people in her house. I have a phone number, so we'll find a phone and call and let her know we're here."

"Appointments for *us*? Are you nuts? I came for the ride!" I snagged Marsha's hand, "I don't want to know any more about what might happen, thank you very much. Just being in my current life is a trial enough, don't you think?"

"Oh, it'll be fun. I'll go first and you can wait for me, if she has time, then you go. If it's terrible or really freaky then you don't have to do it."

"Well," I glared at Marsha from under my eyelids. "As long as you go first. I'll bet she can't see us both."

We got our drinks and found a phone booth in the hotel lobby. The medium could see us both that afternoon after lunch.

The house stood on a slight embankment overlooking a small lake within walking distance of the town. Marsha rang the doorbell while I lingered behind, checking out the scenery around the bungalow. The house seemed to have begun as a camp of sorts perched over the water. A dock with two white Adirondack chairs reached out into the lake and an anhinga lounged on a dead tree drying its wings.

The door opened to a slight, middle-aged woman wearing a simple skirt of flowered cotton, a blue, short sleeved blouse neatly tucked in the skirt and bare legs ending in navy Keds sporting clean white laces. Rosy blush dotted her pale cheeks and a smear of pink lipstick finished her mouth. Arresting brown eyes above a small nose were ringed with fine wrinkles and puffy, greying hair formed a soft cloud about her face. The faint fragrance of an old fashioned perfume clung to her. Needless to say, her appearance was unexpected. I'd imagined a more hipster, Gracie Slick vibe.

"Hello, so good to see you," she reached out her hand to Marsha. "I'm Hazel West Burley. Do come in, it's so warm outside today." Motioning to a small sitting room, she added, "We'll be meeting in here."

Marsha spoke, "I'm Marsha and I'll be seeing you first." She gestured to me. "Kathy is going to see you after I'm finished."

"That is if there's time," I tentatively ventured.

The woman smiled. "Of course. If you'd like to wait for your friend you can sit on the porch. It's fairly cool out there with the breeze and the fans turned on."

She led me to a screened porch fronting the lake. An old swing hung from the rafters and green wicker rockers lined up facing the water. Books were piled high on a rickety table and curious, I surveyed their titles, Edgar Cayce, Alan Watts and others. Not the usual selection one would expect from a woman who looked like someone's maiden aunt. I told myself not to be such a skeptic and settled in to the comfortable worn cushion on the swing. It was breezy out here and strangely not at all hot. Closing my eyes, I let the quiet sink in, the fan stirring the warm, moist air. I must have drifted off because in what seemed like a few minutes, I heard Marsha calling my name.

"Kath, wake up. It's your turn."

"Huh?" I shook my head and opened my eyes to see Marsha standing in front of me.

"Go on in, Hazel is ready for you."

"I guess I fell asleep. It was so weird. How long were you with her?"

"About an hour. You really were sleeping."

"Yeah, I was. I just sat down and the next thing I knew I heard you call my name." I rubbed the back of my neck and shrugged my shoulders. "What was it like?"

"She is amazing. Not weird, just, well... you'll see. I'll be here when you're done. I'll try not to sleep."

I wandered into the house and entered the sitting room. No one was there. Just as I began to sit down in the middle of the sofa, Hazel came in.

"I thought you looked tired so I suggested the porch. It's a special place to doze, there are no dreams."

Speechless, I stared at her.

She gestured to the couch, "I'd like you to sit at this end of the sofa, but first please give me your hands." Facing me, she reached out both hands and grasped mine in a firm grip. Her voice was soft and melodious, "I'm glad you are here." Looking directly into my eyes, she remarked and smiled gently, "Your colors are brilliant." I realized she didn't mean my clothes. She let go of my hands and said, "Sit, please."

Hazel sat at the opposite end of the sofa beside an end table with paper and more books. The room was quiet except for the soft hum of the fan, the breeze over my head cool. A table lamp glowed, though the day outside was still bright and from the windows, I could glimpse the lake with the late afternoon sun glinting off the water.

I glanced at Hazel, who was holding a small linear stone which she rolled between her fingers, her eyes closed. She stopped moving the crystal, dropped it into her lap and opened her eyes. Reaching over, she handed me a piece of paper and a pen, "Please write your name and anything else you choose. I'd like a sample of your handwriting. Not much, just about half a page."

I wrote my name and a brief paragraph describing the room and gave her back the paper. She looked at me as she ran her fingers over the writing.

"You live through much in your unconscious, your dreams. This helps you heal. I see that you are creative and a good teacher. You are a teacher of teachers. And are also strong and possess a great courage." She paused and laid the paper down on the sofa beside her, "Your children will benefit from this. They need you and raising them can be a full time job." She continued, gazing at me, "You are married, yet there is something about the quality of the union and at the same time a caring." She closed her eyes and sighed, picking up the stone and turning it over and over as she swayed back and forth. She opened her eyes and went on, "It is murky. Is this correct?"

I nodded.

"There is more. Could your husband be ill?"

"Yes," I answered, my voice registering surprise.

Hazel didn't respond immediately, then, continued, "You have a great love."

"My husband?"

"No," she said, her voice gentle. "Your husband is very sick."

"My husband is dying."

"Yes, I know. I don't usually tell people these things. It is not for them to know, but you know already. I feel like he does not have long on this earth. You are not with him."

"No, I haven't lived with him for almost year now."

Hazel's hand encircled the quartz stone lying in her lap. Again, she closed her eyes and rocked gently back and forth, sighing and rubbing the stone. She began, eyes still closed, her voice like a chant, "You have journeyed far, many times over and have lost much. Have slept with the dead and burned their Plague riddled corpses. You survived. At times you crawled on your belly and hid in caves. Other times you have removed arrows from your wagon and traveled in the black darkness to avoid the intense heat. Your current journey will take you to the last hilltop where a verdant valley stretches out before you, with paths in many directions. But you must remain on the hillock for some time, your life in limbo. Eventually, you will move on. The path you select will be the right one. Your journey has prepared you well for what lies ahead."

She stopped talking, letting the stone drop in her lap and opened her eyes, taking in deep breaths and turning her head side to side.

Speechless and overwhelmed, I stared at the woman.

Finally she spoke, her voice normal now, low and comforting. "My dear, you and your children are fine and will thrive, but your husband...." She shook her head softly and emitted a barely audible moan, "Oh, your husband has so little time, so little time to make peace." She shuddered. "I fear. I feel fear for him, and I fear for his immortal soul. I'm not sure what has happened, but the spirits are aware of his pain and of his great, great anger."

I sat frozen. The only sound in the room the gentle whirring of the ceiling fan. When I could finally speak, my voice trembled, "My husband is dying of AIDS. He risked my life and our children's. We don't have the virus, we're healthy. I have to believe that we really are, but I feel like the arrows you talk about have pierced my body and my soul." Hazel moved down the sofa taking both my hands into hers.

"Dear, you are well as are your children. Your ancestors have seen to that. They have protected you. You are fine. You will not always be waiting on the precipice. Your next journey will be full, as they always will be and have been. And you have had many journeys over many lifetimes. You will love again, deeply and you will thrive. The spirits, your ancestors, and those not yet spirits will aid you and protect you. They have and will continue to do so." She paused, "Tell me, your father is not spirit but there is something?"

"Yes," I drew in a breath, not believing what I was hearing. "My father had a massive heart attack when I was thirteen. Technically, he died. He had one of the near death things you read about, the tunnel, the white light, but he wasn't ready to go. I was young and my mother and I needed him. He came back and lived and remembered it all. He doesn't talk about it. Thinks people will think he is weird. He's very spiritual, religious and a true Christian."

Still gripping Hazel's hands, I looked into her ancient, kind eyes. "This has all been horrible on my folks. My husband was like a son to them. When I told them about the deception and how my husband lied they were so shocked. They haven't forgiven him, at least not yet."

"Yes, it is so difficult to understand the dark side when most of us confront ours infrequently. Usually our conscience and remorse kick in and we are forced to look and reassess no matter how ugly it may be. This seems to be the checks and balances in the healthy personality. However, as you know, not all are healthy." She paused, "Of course, we want them to be, especially those we care about and spend time with."

The conversation halted momentarily while we sat with our thoughts.

After a brief time, I asked, "You said I would have a great love. Could it have happened already?"

"I don't know. I do know that he will be a friend. Someone with whom you have a friendship first."

"I've fallen in love with a man, a much younger man, but he's left and I think of him constantly and believe that I may always love him."

"Yes," she replied, squeezing my hands and letting go. "You probably will. But he needed to go. Your paths are separate now but will cross again many times, if not in this life, then in others, as has happened in the past. He has much to do, and I think that he needed to leave you to do it all. Is that right?"

"I think. It's just been so hard for me to accept."

"He's younger and needs to prove himself to himself."

"I know that here," I touched my head. "But I don't know why here." I pointed down to my heart.

"Don't doubt his love for you. We can't know in our hearts because it is so painful. As I've said your paths will cross again. Our angels do not ever really leave."

"But in the meantime, what do I do? I'm so sad and it doesn't go away. He's still as much on my mind as he was the day he left."

"And you are also in his. You must feel that. I'm sorry that I don't have an answer for you. I do know that you must wait and be." She patted my hand and stood up. "Your friend has been patient. Our time is up and she has not slept. I hope that I have helped a bit." She smiled down at me, "You can come back anytime."

"Oh, yes, thank you." I got up and reached for my bag. "I owe you money for all this time." Shocked, I realized that we'd been together for over an hour. The afternoon sun was beginning to fade on the water.

"I know money is hard for you now. It won't always be. Can you afford $40?"

Of course she would know that too. "Is forty enough for all our time?"

"For now, it is plenty. But that too will pass. Remember to trust those who are dear to you, particularly those who are noble and have heart."

Chapter 18

My scientific mind stewed over the uncanny pronouncements Hazel had made. It was all too much that she seemed to know those things and still, even skeptical as I was, I couldn't seem to shake what she'd mentioned. My dreams, all that Plague stuff, and as much nonsense as it appeared, the idea that I'd lived other lives. All of it kept coming back to me and the ancestor stuff about protecting me. What was that all about? I wasn't infected, nor were the kids. This was before anyone suspected that there might be a genetic link to HIV. And how would Hazel know anything about that? It all just defied any logical explanations.

As Marsha put it on the ride home, "It isn't about science, it's about faith."

Lucy, back from her rock star travels (she'd spent her seventh birthday riding in a limo around the Eiffel Tower) wanted to stay in Boston with Daddy instead of coming home for the short time before we all went north. She continued to beg and though I wanted her with me I caved. In a way it made sense. Selfishly, the long car ride to Boston would be easier with just one child. Jake and I had fallen into an easy routine; day camp in the mornings while I went into the office or fiddled around at home and most afternoons, at the pool or if it was insufferably hot, we got movies and stayed inside out of the heat.

At work one morning, the phone rang. I was surprised to hear it was Dr. Hal Jacobsen calling to check on me. We chatted for a bit, and I ended up asking him to dinner the next night. Loren was back in town from her vacation and I knew she'd be glad to hang with Jake. Hal happily agreed and we settled on the small French place down the road. I'd meet him there.

Stepping in to the darkened space, my eyes adjusting I looked around. He was at a table, talking with the owner, an older French woman. He'd shaved off his ruddy beard, and without it he looked so different I hardly recognized him. Glancing my way, he stood and smiled.

"It's good to see you." He held out his hand.

"Well, you too." I smiled back taking his hand. "I'm still so grateful to you."

"I'm glad I could be of some help." He hesitated, "How's your husband?"

"He's doing all right. He's in Boston."

"That's right, I remember he was from Boston, had family there, I think."

"Good memory." I nodded. "He does have family there. He actually went back for a number of reasons," I stammered, not sure of what to say next.

"Well, the medical care will definitely be more state of the art than it is here. And you and your children are doing well."

"We are. My daughter is in Boston with Mark, and my little boy and I are going in the next week or so. We'll be there till school starts down here in September."

The owner came for our drink orders, sharing with me that Dr. Jacobsen had saved her life. We sipped a decent red wine as we talked about the menu, the specials and the summer heat in Central Florida. Both of us had grown up in Florida, so we laughed about the Yankees' being babies. Hal, a good listener, drew me out and before I knew it I was telling him the sordid tale of Mark's deception. He seemed not surprised, never flinched, just asked a few pointed questions.

"I figured there was more to it than we'd been told, but there wasn't any reason to go there."

"You think all the doctors knew? " I asked, staring off into the night.

"Probably."

"So, they knew he was lying?"

"Yeah. We don't know that much about the virus as yet, but we do know that it usually shows up within a few years after infection. He may have been HIV positive for a while. We're also beginning to think there may be some people who are genetically immune."

I shook my head thinking I'd misheard him. If Mark had been exposed at some time prior to last year, then why was I okay? I hesitated for a moment, then, decided to share my visit to Casadega and the information about 'ancestors protecting me'. When he didn't respond with a quick smirk, I went on talking about the Plague and my dreams that the medium seemed to know about. At this point, I figured if he didn't assume I was really unhinged, then he must be a trifle off too.

"Genetically immune?" I questioned.

(http://www.hivplusmag.com/research-breakthroughs/2016/3/23/anyone-immune-hiv)

"No one's sure yet. *(Remember, this is 1990)*. It'll take years before we know more and the current research is real spotty, but there seem to be some people," he hesitated, "people kind of like you, who were probably exposed, but who don't get infected. All of this is still conjecture."

"So, these stories of people being infected years ago and then finding out they have it are not true."

"Usually not." He paused, "Could be, but it's unlikely."

"Me being tested when I was, makes the test pretty accurate."

"Yep," he nodded. "You're the one who needs to be careful. You know you are all right, so be sure you find out about anyone you become intimate with."

I smiled wistfully, "Well, that's not an issue right now."

He leaned over and said softly, "Well, it will be at some point." He stopped and took a deep breath. "You are an interesting, bright woman and any man would be crazy not to want you. You husband was a fool."

"It's good it's dark out here. I think I'm blushing Dr. Jacobsen."

"I'm really serious about all that."

A moment of silence passed between us.

"Well, okay." I sighed. "Now, I have a serious question for you, doctor. It's nosy, but what the hell, you know all about me, and I know virtually nothing about you, except you shaved off your beard and have a strong chin." Smiling, I hesitated before continuing, "You haven't mentioned a wife or significant other. And you have photos of children in your office."

"Yep, recently divorced. Two kids." His voice trailed off. "It's tough." A moment passed. He reached over and squeezed my hand. "It's late. I've got hospital rounds in the morning. Thank you for suggesting this and for a nice evening."

"I'm so glad it worked out. And dinner is on me, so don't even begin to argue."

We walked to our cars, and Hal bent down and gave me a chaste kiss, "Good night. Thank you again."

Driving home, I realized there were good people in the world, and this man was one of them. As I went into the house, I still couldn't shake the genetic thing. What if something like that was true?

After seeing Loren out, I walked into the kitchen to shut out the lights and noticed the message light flashing.

Lucy's voice giggled, with the exciting news of her day. They'd sailed, dug for quahogs, and taken the jeep to the end of Duxbury beach and she and Daddy couldn't wait for me and Jake to come *home*. Then, a pause. "I love you. Oh, this is your daughter, Lucy Hayes. Bye."

I glanced at the clock on the wall, 10:30 and dialed Mark's number, preparing to leave a message when he answered, his voice groggy.

"Hello."

"Hi, it's me. Hope I didn't wake you. You sound asleep."

"No, I only sleep a little these days." He sighed, "I took a sleeping pill finally. It hasn't kicked in yet."

"Well, I got Lucy's message and wanted to remind you that I'm driving, not flying because I need a car." She stopped. "Remember, I'm going to the Cape and to Vermont to see folks."

"When did you decide that?"

"I told you that a few days ago."

"Well, I don't remember you telling me anything about it."

"Mark, I've made plans to visit Olivia and Karen. It will give you and both children time to be together."

"I'd have thought you'd miss seeing your daughter, but I guess yucking it up with your friends is more important."

I slammed my hand down on the counter. "You know better than that!"

"Please, spare me your histrionics. You don't want to stay with me. At least be honest."

"You know, I'm not having this conversation. Tell Lucy I'll call tomorrow."

"Just wait a minute, don't hang up," Mark interrupted, his combative edge gone. "Will you stay here if I stay somewhere else?"

"Of course. I'd planned to stay there. You said the Cambridge apartment is open."

"Yes, it's okay for the rest of the summer and most of fall. Alan will be back and forth after Labor Day, and he thinks it's good to have someone in the place."

"I'm still going to drive because I want a car."

"Whatever, do what you want," Mark countered, exasperated. "It'll be a long drive with Jake."

"It'll be fun. We're treating it as an adventure," I replied, determined not to engage in another battle. "Listen, be sure to tell Lucy I called and I'll call again tomorrow. We leave here on Sunday and will call from the road. Goodnight. Hope you can get some sleep."

"Yeah, me too. Good night."

Just as I hung up the phone, it rang. I picked it up on the first ring, expecting Mark's tired voice. "You forget something?"

"Not that I know of, but I am a forgetful kind of guy," Sam's teasing voice crackled over the distance.

We chatted about his work, and I filled him in on my plans for the rest of the summer. "I'm all right. I leave for Boston next Sunday. Jake and I are driving."

"That's what you said in your letter, and you're staying on the Cape and then off to Vermont. That should be really nice and a good break for you."

"Well, not exactly. There's been a change of plans. I just hung up with Mark," I offered reluctantly. " I'm staying at our house." I continued in a rush, "Before you say anything, Mark is moving out to his friend Alan's apartment. It's vacant till Alan gets back sometime this fall."

"If that works for you. Just be careful. Mark's not exactly the most trustworthy guy, but I'm not telling you anything you don't already know." He paused, "I thought you were looking forward to the hanging out in Vermont and on the Cape."

"I was, but then I feel bad not staying with the kids. Lucy has been gone for such a long while."

"But you had planned to have them with you in Vermont for part of the time, hadn't you?"

"I had, but this is better. We'll just be in Vermont less time." I hesitated, "It is really. Mark actually offered to move."

"Hey, enough stuff. I really called cause I wanted to hear your voice and tell you that I miss you."

"And I miss you too. It's so different with you not here. I'm somehow just not as good with you not in my life."

"And I have a huge gap in mine. Work here is wonderful and exciting, I'm now functioning as the village medical authority, so you know how hard up this place is. But even with all that, it's less without you. Look, I know it's late and I know you have to rise and shine for Jake. Say good night to me like I was there."

"Good night, Sam."

"Good night, sweet dreams."

Early the morning, the shrill jangling of the phone startled me awake. It was Marsha with the news that we hoped we'd never hear. The college had lost the suit in federal court and would close its doors in its current location. We'd just celebrated our first graduation and were working toward full accreditation. The shutdown meant students who had not graduated would need to find other programs, and we were all without jobs. The trustees, parents, licensing board (State Board of Independent Colleges and Universities), and Marsha were frantically searching for new space, but it was unlikely that we'd have anything up and running by September. College parents, a supportive county commissioner, the editor of the local paper and various community leaders were working on our behalf, but finding classroom, office, housing and dining space was a huge challenge.

I threw on my clothes, got Jake up and off to day camp and barreled into my office. I was devastated and it was up to me to contact all faculty members, especially those who were gone and may not have heard. We were a small faculty, and a close team. All we'd accomplished out the window. This place had provided a safe haven for students who never thought they'd make it in college and for some it was their only option. Thank goodness, most of the students were gone.

As concerned as I was about the future of the college, this also meant that my somewhat settled life was facing a tailspin. Elbows resting on the familiar desk, I put my head in my hands, closed my eyes and watched as all the awful scenarios marched across my consciousness. I had no job; there were no other jobs in this sleepy little town; I'd have to move back to our house in Boston; we'd need to sell the Florida house, which we'd bought a couple of years ago just to have a place to live near the college, and then, the final overarching realization that maybe, this was all the way it was supposed to be and it was meant for me to go back. Breathing in deeply, I said a silent prayer and asked for strength and more wisdom than I currently possessed.

Chapter 19

The Florida house sold quickly and what furniture I didn't want I left. Mark had willingly taken charge of the moving arrangements, so all I had to do was load the car with things I didn't plan to ship, pack up Jake's and my stuff and hit the road. The movers would do the rest and I'd be in Boston in a week or so. There was hope that something would happen with the College, but no guarantees. After tearful goodbyes to Marsha, colleagues, and the church nursery school folks, Jake and I began our extended road trip north. We stopped at my parents and spent the night. I promised to call daily from the road. This move was difficult for them to grasp, but I needed to try it out since other options were limited. I was determined to remain upbeat.

It was late afternoon, four long days after leaving Florida. Frazzled and dead tired, I'd forgotten about the Cape traffic in the summer on the road out of Boston. Finally, I pulled into the driveway of our weathered antique home, about 25 miles south of the city, and the memories rushed, flooding over anything else I was feeling. This was where we had brought our babies home, where we resurrected the primitive beauty of a circa 1719 lived in home. The granite wall that Mark built stood imposing, clothed with summer sweet pea blossoms. My herbs thrived, the mint tumbled over the border, its fragrance perfuming the warm breeze coming off the pond; and my favorite tree of all, the giant willow, its welcoming arms arched over the water shading the area as it had done for over a century. When we bought the place, I declared I would only leave in a pine box, on my way to the great beyond, heaven, nirvana or somewhere not on this immediate earth.

We were barely out of the car, when Lucy bolted out of the screen door. "Mommy, Jake!" Jake dashed out and into Lucy's arms as she swaddled her brother in a bear hug.

Bending down I picked up Lucy and smothered her face with kisses taking in her sweet little girl scent and nuzzling my face in her tousled hair.

At the sound of feet shuffling, I glanced over and saw Mark walking slowly down the driveway.

"Daddy!" Jake yelled and ran to Mark who squatted down and grabbed him tightly.

The change in Mark's appearance was staggering. His face gaunt, deep grey circles under the piercing blue eyes, his clothes hanging on a skeletal frame. My voice catching, I tried not to show my shock. I forced a lightness I didn't feel.

"Glad you finally got here. She's been waiting all day," he smiled. With a visible effort, he straightened up. "God, has he grown."

Eager to go in, Jake pulled on Mark's hand, "Come on guys, let's go in. I wanna see my room and go in the tepee."

Lucy slid out of my arms and acting as the knowledgeable big sister, took Jake's hand. "Hold my hand cause you don't know where to go. Come on."

I turned to Mark. "I'll get the bags, you go on in with them. We can unpack everything later."

"I can still manage. I'm just thin, not totally disabled."

"I didn't mean." I stammered.

"I can look in the mirror. I still have my sight and I know how I look."

"I'm sorry." I apologized. "It's just that I haven't seen you in a while I guess."

"Yeah, well it's what happens." He stopped. "Open the back and I'll get some of this."

After a few trips, we had unloaded, and I was emptying my suitcase, putting stuff in the closet when Mark came into the bedroom and suggested we eat out, which was fine with me. Silently, I wondered when he was going to the apartment in Cambridge, but didn't want to push it.

I got the kids ready for bed, did tuck-ins, and when I came downstairs, noticed that Mark had fallen asleep on the sofa. Not having the heart to wake him, I covered him up and turned out the lights.

As the morning sun peeped in, I woke up. Mark was sleeping on the far side of the king size bed. I got up, went into the kitchen to make coffee and debated getting him up. Walking outside, I picked up the Boston Globe from the driveway and took my coffee out to the terrace. I had just finished the first section when I heard rumblings in the kitchen.

Mark emerged, coffee in hand and joined me outside. "God, I needed that sleep," he sat down in the opposite chair. "I feel 100% better than I did yesterday."

"Good, you look better. Less tired."

"Yeah, some days are not so good, others more like normal." He took a sip of coffee. "Anything interesting in the paper?"

"It's summer, the city sleeps." I got up. "I'm making toast, want any?"

"Nope, just coffee and then my menu of drugs." He smiled. "What do you and the kids want to do today?"

I stopped in the doorway and looked at him, "Well, I hadn't gotten that far." I paused. "Maybe the beach or the water park. What are your plans?"

"I'm game for anything, you decide," he answered, not looking up from the paper.

I turned and went into the kitchen. I didn't want to create a scene, but was troubled at his automatic assumption that we would spend the day together. And I wondered when he was moving to town, so I called out to him from the kitchen, asking if he needed help with his move.

When he didn't answer, I figured he hadn't heard so I repeated the question as I took my toast outside.

Mark glanced up from the paper and raised his eyebrows, "No, I don't need help."

"Oh, so you must not be taking much."

"Nope. Not anything."

I swallowed the dry lump of toast stuck in my throat and reached for coffee to wash it down.

"I'm not taking anything because I'm not going. It fell through."

Frowning, I put the cup down on the table, "But, that's not what we agreed on."

"Well," he replied evenly and laid the paper down. "Things change. You're here with no other house. No job." He stopped and looked at me, "There's plenty of room here for us all. We did fine last night. It was nice. And, it's a lot easier on the kids."

The next few days went by quietly, the beach healing for me and fun for the children. We grilled hotdogs at night, went for ice cream, and to any outside observer appeared like one happy middle class family relishing the New England summer. Mark and I didn't engage much, and whenever we did,

I purposely kept it light. At night, there was a huge element of uncomfortableness as he crawled into the bed. He slept fitfully and after two nights of being kept awake, I bunked in with Lucy.

After dinner towards the end of the week, I called my friends in Vermont. "Of course you can still come and bring the kids too," Karen's insistence reassured me. "We're looking forward to having you and you can stay as long as you like. The small house down the hill is empty and all yours."

Karen had started a B&B in Vermont when her girls were young so she could stay home with them. Their house was a sprawling Victorian with the upstairs used for guests and recently they'd purchased a small bungalow nearby for larger groups. The B & B turned into a grand venture for her because the money she brought in was extra, and when she didn't want to fool with guests she just put out the no vacancy sign. In her other life, she was a successful artist and a Vermont state representative. Her husband, Warren was a local businessman.

"Are you sure this is not putting you out?" I pressed. "I'm so sorry about all this mess."

"The only thing that is putting me out is Mark. I feel really sorry for him, but still can't believe that he would act like this, but then again I can't believe he did what he did!" She paused to take a breath. "Anyhow, be careful. You know how bad the traffic crawling north can be. We'll see you all for supper."

I hung up the phone and sat on the edge of the bed listening to the children's chatter and the drone of the TV coming on in the living room. Determined to avoid another scene with Mark, I got up and started putting a few things into the suitcase.

Going out into the living room, I plopped down on the sofa next to Lucy and pulled her close. Forcing a cheery note in my voice, I announced that in the morning we were going to Vermont for a while.

Lucy looked up at me, a confused frown on her face, "It's too soon to go there."

Jake whirled around from his position on the floor while the TV continued to fill the room with noise. "I don't want to go back in the car. I'll throw up again"

"Besides, Daddy said we could go to camp and go sailing," Lucy added, quickly ducking out of my embrace.

"Camp doesn't start right away and we'll have fun in Vermont. Let's get your jammies on and then, I'll help you pack." I reached out to take Lucy's hand as she jerked away.

"But I don't want to go. I want to stay here," Lucy insisted, her small chin jutting up in a gesture of defiance.

"Me, either!" Jake chimed in, not turning from the repetitive television.

I responded firmly that we were going and it was time for bed. I'd pack for them if they didn't want to help.

Jake asked if Daddy was going too as he hopped up and bounced to the sofa, shoving over the pillows to sit snug up to Lucy.

Out on the terrace, Mark had overheard the conversation. He came into the room. "I'm not going this time. It's just you and your mother." He stood, arms crossed in front of his chest, a thin smile disguising his disdain. "She seems to think that it's too crowded here."

"I don't think it's crowded," Lucy added.

"Me, either, there's just us," Jake seconded, wriggling closer to his sister.

I stared hard at Mark, my mouth set in a tight line, why was I not surprised? Calmly, I told the kids that we had planned to go to Vermont anyhow, it was just a bit sooner than we thought. And underscoring, in my upbeat voice, Karen had said we could all sleep in the new treehouse.

Jake jumped off the sofa and rushed past me heading for the bedroom. "C'mon Lucy, we can sleep in the treehouse tomorrow if we sleep here now."

Lucy sat still and glanced at her dad. She hung her head down and not speaking, fiddled with her toes.

I moved to go to her, but Mark held up his hand. He sat down beside our small daughter and put his hand on her knee. "Baby, go on with Mommy. She and Jake haven't seen you for a long time and they missed you. I'll be up in a week and get you and Jake for camp. Then, we can all stay here."

"But it's not what I want to do!" Lucy jerked her head up and spun around angrily.

Grinning at her, Mark said, his voice laced with sarcasm, "Well, sweetie your mother has her mind made up."

Pale with anger I smiled back, resolving, not to be engaged. "As Daddy said, I missed you so much and you and Jake can still go to camp."

A pout fixed on her freckled face, Lucy questioned, "Daddy will you be lonely without me?"

"Always, baby, but it's just for a little time." Leaning over he kissed the top of her head. "And think how lonely Mommy was without you when you were here." He paused, "Now go get ready for bed and get some stuff ready to go."

Lucy reluctantly got up from the sofa. Reaching out, I gently patted her on the back. "I'll be there in a minute. See what Jake's up to."

I stood still and glowered at Mark.

"As you see, our daughter also has a mind of her own."

"She's a child!"

"She is a child. But she isn't stupid."

"You set this all up, didn't you? You set me up." Caught up in it all, I snapped at him, my voice breaking.

Mark looked up, the smile leaving his face. "You set yourself up. You don't want to stay here and so you screw it all up and make your daughter miserable. It's always what you want."

"I'm not doing this with you. You went back on your agreement. You were the one who said you'd move out. You were the one who offered. You lied, just like you've lied all along!"

"You're right, I lied. So kill me," he replied. "It'd actually be preferable to the way I'm dying now."

I stopped and took a deep breath, angry and sad at the same time.

Mark propped his head back on the sofa cushion and closed his eyes. When he spoke, the fight was gone from his voice. "Listen," he began, as he opened his eyes. "I want to be with our children. I don't know how long I have to be with them." He paused, "I don't think you want to keep them from me, and I don't think that's what this is about."

I started to speak.

"Let me finish," he continued, "I'll come get them in a week. That's when camp starts. They're signed up for two weeks of camp. You stay in Vermont until you're ready to leave and go to the Cape or wherever. You'll end up back here anyway since the college is kaput. "

Not wanting to open any more wounds, I wanted to choose my words carefully, so I waited for a moment and paced back and forth in front of the sofa. "Mark, it's a lot taking care of two little kids. Jake can be a handful. He's full of energy and doesn't sit still for long. Lucy is," I paused, "well, you know how Lucy is, you've been with her for a couple of months. She's pretty easy, physically, that is, compared to Jake."

"I know Jake takes a lot of energy. But I want to be with my son for as long as I can." He leaned forward and stared hard at me. "I love my children" he paused, "and I still love you."

Not having a response, I looked up at the ceiling and closed my eyes. No one spoke.

Mark broke the silence, "You know, I don't give up easily. I'll do whatever I can to get you back."

I opened my eyes and faced him. "I know that you want it all back the way it was. But it can't ever go back. What we had, you destroyed by what you did. It could have killed us all." I stopped. "I can't just forget that and go on, like it didn't happen."

"I know that. And I'm sorry. But you all are okay, you aren't dying," he said quietly, pain evident in his speech. "I am." He waited to let the words sink in. "I am dying and I want to be with my family. Why is that so difficult to understand?"

"It's not hard to understand, Mark." I glanced out at the cloudless, inky sky, the full summer moon reflecting off the pond. "You could live near us. If the college is resurrected then, we could go back to Florida. If not, we'll stay here. Your travel schedule is full so you come and go anyway." I hesitated and went on. "There'll probably come a time when you won't be able to work and will need help. We have friends and family in both places and good doctors here and in Florida. Dr. Jacobsen is a good man and knows people. We can all help. I can help."

Mark said nothing for a moment. He sat still, gazing past me. When he finally spoke any vestiges of conciliation were gone. "You know, I wouldn't have left you because you had AIDS, but then," he reflected, his eyes meeting mine, "but then, I've never been so swayed by a young lover."

I said nothing, attempting to quell the mounting rage as my eyes trailed over his spent body and finally settled on his thin, pallid face. He was in such pain and so tormented that when I finally spoke, I was even and controlled. "You know I didn't leave you because you had AIDS. I left you because you lied to me, to everyone. You betrayed my trust. I went for months not knowing if our children were going to die, not knowing if I was going to die. You risked my life and our children's lives by having unprotected sex with random people.

You knew the risk!" I swallowed hard trying to control my quivering voice. "You repeatedly say you love us and yet you did that. You played fucking Russian Roulette and you lost. By the grace of God we didn't." I was on the verge of tears and not wanting him to see me cry, I turned and started out of the room, when I felt his viselike grip on my shoulder.

"I won't let you take my children from me. You can do what you want with whomever you please, but I will not lose my kids," he hissed, his face close, his warm, sickly breath sticky on my face.

"Take your hand off me!" I jerked back pulling away. "I have no intention of taking your children away, but I will not be blackmailed by you."

Suddenly, Mark stumbled away, clutched his chest and began to cough. Taking out a clean handkerchief, he held it to his mouth while the hacking wracked his emaciated frame.

I started over to him, but he waved me away. The coughing subsided, and he removed the handkerchief. It was streaked with blood.

I reached out to touch his arm.

"Don't." He shook his head, tears in his eyes from the coughing fit. "It passes and I'm used to it. I have a breathing treatment at the end of the week, then I'm good to go for a month or two."

Covering my mouth with my hand, my eyes filled with tears.

"So," Mark said and wiped his brow where sweat had formed from the force of the coughing. "I'll be up to get both kids in a week for camp. After that we'll go from there."

Chapter 20

The days spent with Lucy and Jake in Vermont passed quickly in a whirlwind of childhood adventures. Both mastered the swim to the float moored in the cold lake and got up at first light to peer down through the canopy of branches from the treehouse perch. They competed in vegetable picking, ate blueberries from the bushes that stained their teeth and about every night we'd stroll or bike ride to town for Ben and Jerry's.

I relished the best of the New England season with a new found appreciation for the life I was given, my overwhelming gratitude coupled with an edge of sadness for what was lost.

Karen, the wise and ever vigilant hostess did everything to boost my spirits and lavished sincere love and praise on the kids. Her girls were older and took my two under their wings, reading, painting, and papering the treehouse with all varieties of kid artwork. Lucy missed Mark but with the busyness of the days, she fell into bed and slept deeply each night. Jake was enamored of all of it, following the girls everywhere and relishing the dirt and fantasy of sleeping in the trees.

Over coffee one morning I reached out and grabbed Karen's hand telling her how much they all meant to me and how thankful I was that she and her husband took me in.

Karen leaned over and rested her head on my shoulder. "I know what you are thinking and not one word out of you. The kids leave this weekend with Mark and you are staying here with us. We love having you in the house. We don't worry when we leave to go to the lake and stay a few days. You work like a housemaid in the B&B, make and buy great food, insist on real cream, feed the dog, laugh at Warren's jokes and pick up your clothes. What better house guest is there?" She smiled up at me and raised her arched eyebrows, "Besides, he is overjoyed he has cream for his 'good' coffee and no one fusses when he scarfs the Ben and Jerry's.

Getting up I put my arms around Karen, hugging her close. "You all are the best friends I could ever hope for. You know you mean the world to me, and I don't know how to thank you for everything you've done."

"And it is mutual. Now that's settled." Karen hesitated. She then moved on to Mark. "Well," she screwed up her face as she got up to get more coffee. "I don't know if I even want to see him. I might tell him off like Patricia did."

I had to smile. My friend Patricia went off on Mark. I'm not sure if it was in person or on the phone, but it seemed like she let him have it.

"Didn't he "un-godmother her or something?" Karen asked me.

"He did!" I laughed and sat back down. "Un-godmothered! That has to be a first, but you know how seriously she takes those church things. She still hasn't stopped talking about it."

"How do you un-godmother someone?"

"Well, he told Patricia that he would have her name removed from the baptismal records in the church, and she believed him."

Just then the phone rang and daughter Amy yelled from the hall, "I'll get it." Then another yell of, "It's Mr. Hayes."

I walked over to the phone on the kitchen wall and picked it up. "I've got it, thanks." I really did not want to engage with Mark, just set a time and leave it. I took a deep breath.

"Hi. Uh huh, the weather's beautiful, warm and sunny. Well, that works. No, I'm going to stay here for a while. I'll get them packed up and we'll see you in a couple of days. Take care. Bye." I replaced the receiver and filled Karen in on the latest developments with the college.

The college had been reestablished and moved to a nearby town. (It is still functioning today, 30 years later, and is thriving.) Marsha wanted me back in late September and it seemed that most of us would return. No word from Sam, he was unsure at this point, but I was ready to go back. I missed having my folks nearby and the 'family' I had in the south. Mark's dad had his hands full with his mom, and his nearby brother's life was busy. It was hard to count on them with all they had on their plates.

I hadn't told Mark that I was going back to Florida. The responsible part of me felt deceptive doing this behind his back, but then the outraged part of me held on to the way he behaved about staying in the house and I knew it was the right decision. My internal conflicts would be living with me for some time.

I'd found a rental house in downtown Mt Dora and both kids would be in the same elementary school; Jake was beginning kindergarten. They would be going home after school on my late days with their former nursery teacher whose family we all knew. It had worked out with grace, serendipity, and genuine concern from the church community who had embraced us and helped set it up.

The following morning I woke early to find Jake snuggled beside me in the old four poster bed. Leaning over I kissed his damp forehead and thought how much I'd miss him with his energy and excitement about life, even for a brief few weeks. He needed to spend time with Mark, but he and I had become such a team with Lucy gone. It would be tough to be without the kids. I figured it was like that for Mark too and my guilt kicked in, but then my resolve overrode it, and I knew what I had arranged was the best for me and the children. Mark was healthy and mobile for now, and he didn't need to be in our old, large house alone either. He could see the children whenever he wanted.

I climbed out of bed and tiptoed down the hall to where Lucy was sleeping. Perched on the edge of the twin bed, I watched my small, serious daughter as she appeared to dream, her eyelids flickering in deep sleep. I hoped her dreams were frivolous and free of worry. She seemed to bear the burdens of the world on her newly turned seven year old shoulders. Bending over, I brushed her cheek with a light kiss.

The next morning, after a full, final Vermont day with the kids, I was upstairs in the guest areas when I heard a car pull into the graveled driveway. I peered out the window and saw Mark standing by his car looking up at the distant mountains. I watched as he turned away, stepped up to the side porch and lifted the knocker, rapping on the door. Someone answered the door, then, voices as Mark came into the house.

Uncertain whom he was talking with, I crept into the hall and crouched over the banister. Warren and Mark stood in the foyer. They spoke quietly and all I could make out was sounds, no words.

Then I heard footsteps clicking on the wooden floor and Karen appeared beside Warren. More inaudible words were mumbled and then Karen's clear, raised voice, telling Mark, "Please, spare me, Mark. This isn't about choosing sides."

Mark shot back with something like he would wait in the car because he wasn't welcome here. He turned away and stormed out, banging the door.

Warren wrapped his arm around Karen who leaned into his shoulder. Wordlessly, they walked together towards the back of the house.

I ventured down the stairs and out to where Mark sat seething in his car. I waved to him in an offhand way telling him the kids were out back with the big girls and I'd get them.

Their excited voices rose from the treehouse as Lucy and Jake clambered down the rope ladder racing each other to be first to Dad's car.

"I won!" I heard Lucy announce in a victorious shout.

"Nuh uh!" Jake yelled back. "Daddy, tell her I was first."

Mark had gotten out of the car when he saw the children running and encircled them both in his arms. He hugged them close. "You know," he grinned, hugging the children close, "I think it was a tie. You both were here at the same time."

I had come around from the garden side of the house and stood still as I watched Mark with the children, a catch in my throat, while they laughed and talked with a dad who would become a memory. He wouldn't be alive to see Lu master tennis or Jake win his first swim meet. I slowed my pace to give them time alone.

"Where's Mommy?" Jake turned toward the back scanning for me.

"She's in the garden, silly. Mommy's fine," Lucy answered in a matter of fact voice. "Daddy," she looked up at Mark, "I'll go get my stuff. Aren't you coming in to see Karen and Warren?"

"I've been in, honey and seen them both. You run and get your things and we'll get on the road. Can you get help Jake get his?"

"I don't need help," Jake insisted, indignant. "I can get my stuff myself. C'mon Lucy. Let's race again."

Lucy glanced over her shoulder at her dad with a look of fragile toleration. "I'll help him," she remarked and turned to Jake. "Okay, you get your bag that Mom packed, and I'll come in and see if anything is left."

I made it to the car just as the kids were hurrying towards the house, delaying before I said anything. This conversation was not one I wanted to have, but I had decided that I was not staying in snowy New England, in our giant, difficult to maintain house, with no job, living with Mark. I shaded my eyes and leaned into the car. "I'm going to stay here while they're at camp and then I'll come into town, probably go to the Cape for a bit. We'll go back to Florida shortly after that. The kids' school starts the last of August and the college will be relocating and ready for classes later in the fall."

Mark said nothing. He stared straight ahead. A moment passed as his gaze wandered past me. Then, he asked me where I planned to live since we had sold the Florida house. When I told him I had a rental in Mt. Dora through church friends, he laughed, reminding me that I had an incredible home on over 7 acres that was free and that I certainly must have lost my mind.

Ignoring his comment I went on. "Well, how are you doing? You look like you feel better."

"I'm okay, figure the new drugs are working. I'm free until September and then we hit the road again."

"The group, they've done so well. I mean, who'd have thought that a bunch of basically, teenagers would have taken over the pop music scene." Uncomfortable, I paused, attempting to maintain a civil conversation.

"I've a piece coming out next month in the Rolling Stone. They're interested in a monthly about being on the road with the band."

I was genuinely happy for him.

"The monthly works out okay because anything long term seems dumb when you won't be around to see it." He cut his eyes to me.

Interrupted by Jake's shrill shriek I looked toward the upstairs window, "Mommy, she won't let me carry my stuff!"

"Mommy, he can't carry it all. He's made a mess," Lucy screamed in the background.

"I'm coming," I shouted up at the window.

A few minutes later, after repeatedly kissing the children, I got them settled in the car, making sure that Jake had the shotgun seat and a damp towel and plastic bag in case he got car sick.

As they pulled away, I stood in the driveway and waved good bye, then strolled back into the house and to the kitchen where Karen was fixing lunch.

"I couldn't help myself. I wasn't kind or charitable or even very nice." Unsettled, she glanced up at me, "I'm just so mad at him for all sorts of reasons!" She smacked down the sharp knife on the butcher block, pulverizing the celery.

"It's all right," I sat down across from her. "We don't have guidelines for how to respond to someone we loved who did something stupid and hurtful and is dying. You shouldn't die for having sex. Someday, this won't happen, but not in time for so many folks."

"You know," She sighed, looking up, the knife suspended, "I never thought of it that way. We did love him. He did something horrible to you, and I'm sorry he is going to die. I guess I just miss who he was to us all." She put down the knife and wiped her hands on the tea towel on the counter. "But why is he such an arrogant ass?"

"Maybe he was an ass all along. Maybe, because he was also so charming and interesting, we didn't care." I shrugged, "Who knows? I knew his history, married him anyway, had his kids, was I such a total fool?"

Karen stepped away from the cutting board. "No, we were all fooled. It wasn't just you. Mark was, and is," she paused, "still seductive, smart, and no one, I mean no one would have guessed that he screwed around for years." She shook her head at me, "No one."

Just then, Warren walked in with a stack of mail, "Hey, ladies, what's for lunch?" He walked over, gave me a squeeze and grabbed Karen around the waist, nuzzling her neck, "My bride, what say we take our lovely house guest to dinner and dancing? There's a live band tonight."

"Live?" Karen wrinkled her nose at him. "That means that there's someone in the group who's only mostly dead."

"Now, now. It's just a matter of time and with luck, we'll be the old geezers," he smiled and deposited a kiss on Karen's cheek. He turned to me, "Kathy Ann there's mail for you. I signed for it. Figured it might be important."

I'd had my mail forwarded to their house, not wanting Mark to see anything from Sam and snoop around. The envelope was from the insurance company. "Good Lord! This says that insurance on the car has been cancelled for nonpayment, and I can't get any more insurance because of the nonpayment." I dropped the paper on the counter and stared at Warren. "This must be a mistake."

Taking the letter, he read silently. "Well," he said, "this says that you didn't respond to the earlier notice and that your insurance was actually cancelled a month ago." He looked at me. "Before you left Florida."

"I didn't get any notice! Before I left Florida? You mean I've been driving the whole time with no insurance."

Warren glanced from me to Karen. "Seems like that."

"Mark pays the insurance on the car and on the house. The bill goes to him in Boston. I didn't see a notice."

"It says that once insurance in Florida is cancelled for nonpayment and you don't respond within a set time, the company cancels and you become an assigned risk," Warren replied. "It's different in each state." He spoke to Karen as he left the room, "I'll call our guy."

"We'll figure it out," Karen tried to reassure me. "Sit there and have a glass of tea while Warren finds out what you need to do."

Just then, the doorbell rang, long and hard.

"Tea's in the refrigerator," she added and went to answer the door.

I got up and was pouring a glass of tea over ice when Karen called me to the door, where a large, burly guy stood. He asked me if I was Kathryn Jarvis. I looked at Karen, then, at the man, "Yes, I am. Why?"

He reached into his shirt pocket and took out a folded document, which he held out to me. "You've been served."

Somewhere in the distance, I heard Karen and Warren talking. She must have gone to find Warren when the man handed me the papers, but it was fuzzy, like I was floating above the floor and watching myself on a stage set. My hands shook as I considered the document. Carefully examining the gummed flap I slipped my nail under the loose corner, tearing it open and read: Mark Hayes v Kathryn Jarvis filed in the District Court of Plymouth County, Brockton, Massachusetts, Petition Seeking Child Custody. The coversheet stated that "the attached is a lawsuit filed by Mark Hayes seeking custody of Lucy Kate and John Thomas." I had 20 days in which to respond to the pleading. Failure to respond would result in a default judgment in favor of the plaintiff.

Scanning the remaining pages, I waded through the legalese and stared in disbelief at the sheaf of papers in my trembling hand. Mark must have known about the college. Suspended in time, I was unaware that Karen and Warren had come back into the hallway. Karen rested her hand on my shoulder and led me into the kitchen. They'd found the phone number for the Boston lawyer who'd helped me with the legal separation and called him for me. He was calling back in a few minutes to help me interpret.

Warren had also taken care of the lapsed car insurance. His agent in Vermont was working with the folks in Florida. It would be expensive for a while but at least I'd be covered.

I looked from Karen to Warren with a grateful thank you and rested my head in my hands, elbows on the counter. I shut my eyes and paused for a moment, then straightened up, fury coursing through every fiber of my being. "What in the hell is he thinking? Mark must be really crazy! First, no car insurance in a vehicle that his kids ride in! And now, custody? Really? No court would give a dying man custody of his kids. And the publicity! If this gets out, Mark's position, oh, dear Lord, the press will have a field day."

Karen and Warren said nothing.

I stared at them, a horrified look clouding my face, "You're not saying anything. Do you think he might have a case?"

Karen sat down beside me and put an arm around my shoulders, "No, no I don't think that; surely a court won't give him custody..." She shifted her eyes to Warren waiting for him to help her.

"Kathy Ann, I don't know what a court will do. Of course, it makes no sense to give custody to someone who is ill, like Mark, but courts behave strangely about custody issues sometimes. You have to be prepared for anything. "

"In the meantime, I need a glass of wine." Karen got up and opened the refrigerator. "Honey," she said to Warren. "Get us some glasses, please."

"My bride, this calls for stronger stuff. He turned to me and raised his eyebrows with a wan smile, "Joining me?"

We took their drinks outside and sat quietly, on the top deck, overlooking the lush garden, the mountains in the far distance. Karen went back inside and brought a Cobb salad she had concocted earlier out to the table. We were putting forks down when the portable phone rang. I took the call.

Briefly, I told the story while my attorney listened. When I finished, there was silence for a moment, then he asked me about money. "You have a lot of money?"

"What?" I questioned, thinking I hadn't heard him correctly.

"Custody battles are some of the most costly legal proceedings," he clarified. "You may have to pay for social workers, psychologists, expert witness folks, in addition to the hours of lawyer fees. You have twenty days to file a response."

I bit my lip and stared down into the empty drink glass. A moment passed before I said anything.

"How much do you need to file a response?"

"Nothing right now, because you're an established client. I'll keep costs down as much as possible, but it's a puzzling case and somewhat complicated. You see, no one has custody of your children because you are still married. Also, the kids have lived in Florida. I know you sold the house, but you are planning to take them back soon for school." He went on, "I don't know why the Commonwealth would entertain the suit since the children and you are domiciled in Florida. We may get lucky."

"So, what are you saying?"

"Well, I'm inclined to file a motion to dismiss for lack of proper jurisdiction. That's our best shot and if that doesn't fly, then I'd suggest that the Commonwealth gives you custody of your children. If you agree, I'll get right on this. You'll still have to show in court, though."

I gave him the go ahead, put down the phone, shoved my chair back and struggled to my feet. The shirt caught on the edge of the chair, ripping, a corner of blue chambray waving in the slight breeze. Apologizing to Karen and Warren, I stumbled and covered my mouth with my hand. Reaching out, I yanked the frayed cloth loose from its vice in the wooden webbing while the heavy chair toppled over, crashing to the deck floor.

Chapter 21

The stupid back button loop on the stupid silk blouse wouldn't fit over the button and the silk blouse was already stuck to my damp body. It was just past 6:00 am, and already, it was a steamy, Cape Cod summer day. I shoved open the bedroom door and stormed down the long hall to Olivia's bedroom. It was empty. Continuing through the hall, I marched down the stairs, my kitten heels slapping on each stair tread. In the kitchen, Olivia and Patricia were talking quietly and looked up when I clomped into the room.

Exasperated, frustrated and just done, already, I fussed that I couldn't get the damned thing buttoned, it was hot, and I looked ridiculous.

"Well, you do look sort of like you're collecting for the Salvation Army," Patricia chuckled, surveying my plain dark silk ensemble.

"Stop it," Olivia shushed Patricia. "She has to look that way in court. She can't go in her short skirt and flip flops. So just hush. Katrina (a fond name she used for me), turn around so I can fix the hook."

Obediently, I shrugged, and turned around, holding my hair off my damp neck so Olivia could do the button.

Olivia looked critically and shook her head, "Your hair will never do. Here, sit down and I'll put it up."

"It'll just fall down!"

"I don't care. Sit."

In a few minutes, Olivia had my hair in a tight chignon, "Now, you look like a prim matron who would never do any of the things Mark could possibly accuse you of."

My eyes shifted from Olivia to Patricia. "Accuse me of what?" My voice rose, "I haven't done anything."

"Don't look at me," Patricia said and took a gulp of coffee. "I just came down at this unfortunate hour to give you moral support. I told Mark off the last time I saw him, and he un-god mothered me." She grimaced, "If he's willing to take on the church who knows what he'll do in court."

"I told her that," Olivia emitted a frustrated sigh and glared at me. "She won't believe me. The man will say anything to get what he wants. Her lawyer has warned her too."

"Please, I've heard it all. I know Mark's a deceitful liar, but I haven't done anything to make a court not give me the children."

"He'll make stuff up and use things that you never think of," Olivia frowned.

I busied myself by pouring coffee into the empty cup on the counter. The steam rose like a fragrant fog and inhaling, I breathed deeply, trying to calm my overwrought mind.

"She's right you know," Patricia raised her eyebrows and nodded her head. "Mark's capable of about anything. Just be ready."

I needed to go. The traffic from the Cape into the Brockton court would be a nightmare, so I kissed both of my dear friends, telling them I'd call when I could, when it was over, hopefully.

By the Sagamore Bridge traffic was snarled, the car sweltering, and when I turned on the anemic air conditioner, the car began to overheat. Great! I glowered at the clock on the dash, it worked, so why not the air? I breathed. Get a grip. I had about an hour and a half to Brockton, then, I needed to park and get to court. It would be close. The damned high necked, silk blouse stuck to me and to the seat, the panty hose Olivia insisted on were suffocating and even though having the windows down brought some relief, my hair was coming out of the tight bun while the slight wind coming off the canal merely teased.

After the bridge, the traffic began to move a bit faster and I kept a steady pace until the back up for the exit. Mark, a true Boston native always knew ways around the constant traffic mess; he'd know how to dodge this. Lately, thinking about Mark only brought sadness, not the rage I wanted to feel at what he was doing to me and the children. 'Stop it!' I chanted to the universe as my mind whirled. 'Yes, he may be desperate and sick, and he is committed to getting what he wants. Do not go there and don't get caught up in feeling sorry for him!'

A few blocks from the courthouse, I spied a parking lot with a few empty spaces, pulled in, gave the attendant my keys and dashed down the street, my hair finally giving up, the 'up do'. I had five minutes until court convened. Running up the granite steps, I heaved open the heavy doors, looked around for a sign to the ladies room when I heard, "Kathryn, come on, we need to go in."

My attorney approached, smiling. "I almost didn't know you! I know I said to dress down and boy, did you! I hoped we would have a minute to chat before..." He surveyed my sweat stained clothes and drooping hair. "So, you must have had traffic?" Touching my elbow, he eased me in the direction of the ladies room. "You have about a minute."

A minute later, my hair shored up, lipstick on, blouse and skirt smoothed out, I emerged.

"Is this all right?" I glanced uneasily down at my skirt.

"Oh, yes, it's perfect for court, just not you, I don't think." He paused and took my arm. "We need to go in. Mark is sitting down front with his attorney, Cynthia Cone. We'll be on the other side of the aisle. Don't say anything or volunteer any information no matter how bad it gets."

"I know. We talked about all this."

"I know we did. It's just that it's different when you're in the courtroom and your husband's lawyer is saying things that may not be true."

I drew in a deep breath, "I will not say one word, no matter how bad it is. I promise."

Once seated on the hard pew like bench, I glanced over at Mark. He could have been the mayor, chatting, smiling and shaking hands as folks he seemed to know, stopped to say hello. His 'rock star' connections went far in this home grown town, where local boys had made them proud. Finally, people moved on to their seats and Mark sat facing forward, his shoulders stooped over in the too big, navy blazer, his head jutting out of the shirt collar, which swam around his stalk like neck.

He had a big head. We'd laughed about that once. He'd claimed his brain took up so much space. I remembered telling him that was 'hokum'. He threw back his giant head, laughing at my choice of words. 'Hokum? Really?' he'd countered. Leaning over to whisper something to his lawyer, he caught me watching him. Embarrassed, I hastily looked away.

The proceedings went along smoothly as the judge questioned both attorneys with what sounded like routine courtroom protocol until Mark's attorney mentioned 'unfit' then proceeded to describe how Ms. Jarvis and her young lover watched dirty movies with her daughter, Lucy, in the room.

Horrified, I grabbed my lawyer's sleeve. He patted me on the arm and shook his head, saying nothing.

The lawyer continued to expound on Ms. Jarvis' affair and clarify that although, Mark had a terminal illness, he was currently in good health and wanted to be with his children for as long as he could. While I listened to this woman talk about me, I looked to Mark for any sign of remorse or acknowledgment that the lies and fantasies being spun affected him in some way. He sat, staring straight ahead, not moving.

The judge said something and my attorney stood up and began. He refuted the charges that Cynthia had leveled and reiterated that Mark was sick and dying of AIDS. He finished with the fact that the children and I were Florida residents, not residents of the Commonwealth, and that the case should be dismissed due to improper jurisdiction.

As he sat down, the judge shuffled the notes in his hand and glanced down. A moment passed while he appeared to consider the papers in front of him. He looked up and directed his gaze to Cynthia as he spoke, "These children appear to be residents of Florida, and this matter should not be settled in this court. There is no need to proceed further in the Commonwealth, therefore, I am remanding this case to the Florida courts."

We all stood and the judge exited the room.

I whispered, "What does this mean for now?"

"You and the children get the hell out of Dodge, leave the state immediately and head home to Florida."

"Now? This afternoon?"

"Yes, as soon as you can get them in the car."

"Why the hurry?"

"Cynthia will have a stop action filed this afternoon if she can and you'll be stuck here and he'll have another shot at this." He took my hand. "The Massachusetts courts are liberal. Florida isn't. He won't have a prayer in the Florida courts and he and Cynthia know it."

"So this isn't resolved. I still have to worry about Mark taking the kids. Is that what you're saying?"

"No, it's not resolved in a court." He hesitated, "But it is resolved in a way. You have the kids, you're their mother, you and Mark are legally separated in Florida and you have been and continue to be the primary, custodial parent."

"I didn't do any of those things that, that woman said I did." I swallowed the building lump and went on, "How can anyone believe all that stuff? How could Mark honestly say these things about me?" Tears welled up.

"It's not about you." He took my arm and began walking me out of the courtroom. "This is about Mark wanting the children. From what you've told me, he's used to getting what he wants." He stopped. "And that is why you are leaving Massachusetts today with your children. It'd be better if you could stay with someone out of state and avoid motels until you get some distance."

"Why?"

"I don't trust your husband not to follow and take the kids or to use the press for his advantage. I saw how he worked the room before court started."

"You're serious?"

"Yep, I'm serious. Right now, we stop by the clerk's office to get paperwork that clarifies the ruling." Looking at my concerned face, he continued, "You'll be fine and I'm just being extra cautious. Relax. It's going to be okay. Really. We won today."

At the nearest gas station, I peeled off the rumpled court attire, threw on a tee shirt, shorts and sandals and checked the time. The children's camp got out about 4:00 and it was just lunchtime. If I hurried I could be there after lunch. First, I had to go to the house and get their stuff. Mark was probably meeting with his attorney and while I wanted to avoid a confrontation with him the kids needed their things.

Fretting about where out of state I could get to tonight, I initially came up blank, then remembered that Mike, our pediatrician friend and his family had recently relocated to Connecticut. It was just over the Massachusetts line right off the turnpike, not a long drive. Mike had been one of the first people I'd called when I found out that Mark had AIDS. Dropping coins into the gas station pay phone, I prayed that someone would be at home.

Within seconds, his wife Ruth answered and I filled her in on court and needing to leave the state. She assured me they'd love to have us. It was no problem and would give us an easy place to rest for the night.

"You come right on. Mike's home early today and the kids will be thrilled to see your little ones. We're just over the Massachusetts line. Get off the

A Red Door

turnpike at the first Connecticut exit, pull into the only gas station there and call us. We'll give you directions from there."

Back in the car, I raced the back roads to our house, dashed up the stairs, grabbed clothes, toys, anything that I knew they'd need and rushed to the day camp, which was by the town center. Once there, I found the counselor who seemed in charge and introduced myself.

"I've come to pick them up early," I hesitated, before going on, "and I'm sorry, but they won't be back. We're going home to Florida."

The young man regarded me, a perplexed expression on his face. "I thought they were here for the rest of the summer. Mr. Hayes mentioned that they would be attending the school here this fall, and I was looking forward to working with them in the after school program."

"Well, there's been a change of plans and I'm here to pick them up."

"Well, all right but they do need to check out," he responded uncertainly. "Give me a minute while I find the camp director."

I realized I shouldn't have said anything about leaving. It was too late now.

The counselor came back frowning, "I'm sorry, but the director needs to see you. It seems Mr. Hayes is with him and waiting for the kids."

Chapter 22

I walked the short distance to the small office in the school building that had been relegated to the camp for the summer, expecting Mark to jump out at any moment, but there was no sign of him yet. No one was at the counter, so I called out and a man's voice responded telling me to come on in. Still no sign of Mark. After a brief introduction, I told him I was here for the children.

From behind me, I heard a raspy, "He knows why you're here."

It was tough not to turn around, but I ignored Mark, opened my purse, took out the court document and handed the paper to the director. "I've a record of the court proceedings from this morning and have been instructed by my attorney to take the children home to Florida."

He looked at me and then at the paper, glancing nervously at Mark. "Let's step into my office where we can sort this out in private"

Mark moved to block the doorway of the office and scowled at me as I maneuvered around him. "This is ridiculous! Rick, you know the children will be here in the fall."

Director Rick sighed and sat down heavily, protected, behind his old school desk. "Mark, this is a court order. I don't have a choice here."

Mark stamped into the office and strode to the desk leaning in, both hands resting on the desk. "Rick, you know me. For god's sake, your kids have come backstage with us. You know this," he tilted his head toward me, "situation."

Eyes on Mark, I spoke, my voice controlled, "Whatever the situation, as you put it, I have a court order here to take our children to Florida, and I intend to act on it." I looked from Mark to Rick. No one said anything.

"Well, then, the police station is just across the square." I turned and marched out of the door.

A hefty, older policeman sat behind a tall desk, and I briefly filled him in. He listened politely, barely looking up, then, gestured to the chairs lined up by the wall. He told me to take a seat, that another officer would be out shortly.

Just when I sat down, Mark barreled in the front door, out of breath and stopped at the desk. "I'm looking for my wife. She came in with some lame story about custody."

The man inclined his head towards me and answered in a flat voice, "Have a seat. An officer will be with you shortly."

All color drained from Mark's face, his hands clenched at his sides, he crossed over to where I sat. He bent down and menacingly snarled, "I'll kill you for this."

Even before I had a chance to register what Mark had said, the policeman was out from behind the desk and at my side. He spoke directly to Mark, "Sir, if you threaten this woman in my presence again, I'll be forced to arrest you."

Mark straightened up and glared at the policeman. He hesitated. Then glowering down at me, his voice cold, he spat out, "Hell will freeze over, I'm warning you." Whipping around, he crashed out of the door.

The policeman sat down in the chair next to me and asked kindly if I was all right. I swallowed, thanking him and explained about the court order.

He waited for a moment and shook his head, his concern evident. "Tragic thing, divorce. You'll be wanting some help to get them, I expect." He paused, "It's not too busy this time of day. I can go, just need some coverage for the desk." With an effort, he stood and looked down at me, "Be back in a minute. You sure you're all right?"

"Yes, I'm okay. My husband is sick and angry, but he's never hit me or anything like that." I smiled weakly, a lump lodging in my throat, "I'll be all right, really. Thanks."

It was lunchtime and all the children were in the school cafeteria, small voices buzzing, chairs scraping the worn floor as kids bounced up and down. Looking around I glimpsed the top of Lucy's sun kissed reddish hair, walked over to where she sat eating and planted a kiss on the back of her head.

"Mommy!" Lucy jumped up and grabbed me around the neck. "When did you get here?" She glanced behind me asking, "And where's Daddy?" Then, she scanned the room, stopped and yelled so her voice could be heard two tables over, "Jake, Mommy's here. Look!" she pointed at me like I was an unusual specimen.

I watched Jake's head bob up and down as he snaked the aisles between the tables. "Mommy!" he shrieked, throwing his arms around my waist.

Kissing him, I squeezed my eyes against the building tears and held him tight.

"Mrs. Hayes, the children should finish their lunch." Opening my eyes, I saw the camp director standing beside the table.

Releasing Jake, I smiled sweetly and told him I'd just get their things.

"I don't want any more lunch. I want to go with Mommy." Jake peered up and in his most endearing voice asked, "May I please?"

I couldn't help but grin at this young child's quick read of the necessary niceties.

Obedient to Director Rick's command, Lucy sat down, picked up her sandwich and said, "I'll finish mine, then go get my stuff. Where are we going?"

"Home, sweetie."

"Back to our house?"

"No, back home, to Florida."

"Florida? But, I don't want to go to Florida. Where's Daddy?" Lucy asked, matter-of-fact, putting down her sandwich.

The director intervened, telling Lucy to finish up and come to his office.

Lucy studied his face, then, gazed up at me.

"Sweetie, you can to take it with you and finish it on the way."

As the four of us left the lunchroom, Lucy saw Mark coming down the hall and bolting, she ran to his arms asking him if he was coming to Florida and if not, then she wasn't going either.

Jake chimed in, "But I want to go to Florida. I want to go home. You want me to go home, don't you Mommy?" Jake looked at me, confused, his blue eyes wide.

"Of course!" I squeezed his hand, reassuring him. "And we are going home. Lucy, too."

"No, I'm not going." Lucy whirled away out of Mark's arms and faced me, "I want to stay here with Daddy. I won't go unless Daddy comes too."

I released Jake's hand and squatted down to face Lucy, "Sweetie, Daddy comes and visits all the time and school starts soon and everyone misses you so much. It's time to go home."

"No, Mommy." Lucy's eyes filled with tears as she reached out over to Mark. "I'm not going. You can't make me go!" She raised her voice and stamped her foot, her face screwed up in an angry frown, tears spilling over.

I hung my head as Jake started to fuss, "Mommy, make her come home. What's wrong?" he glanced uncertainly from Mark to me, "Mommy, it's okay," he reached out and put his hands on my head.

Raising my face I kissed Jake and stood up, fixing Mark with a steely stare. "Lucy, I'm getting your stuff and Jake's. The car is outside and it's time to go. Your dad can bring you out to the car."

"See, she doesn't want to go," Mark said, a smug grin playing at the corner of his mouth. "You can take her out to the car."

Open mouthed, I stared at him in disbelief. Pollyanna, that I was, it was finally dawning on me that he would do anything, including using the children, to get what he wanted. Standing silently, I saw the policeman walking quietly down the hall to where we stood.

As he approached, the director, who'd been a silent witness to this mess, spoke up, "May I help you, officer?"

"No, just came on in to see if this lady," he gestured to me, "needs any help."

Jake and Lucy peered up at the policeman.

"Mommy, why do you need help?" Jake asked.

Lucy clung to Mark.

Putting my arms around Jake, I told him it was fine and that the policeman was just checking on us. I paused and told the officer it was taking a bit longer.

"Well, can I do anything to help?" he asked, as he eyed Mark.

Mark glared back and picked Lucy up, "I was just saying goodbye to my children."

The director hurried off to get the children's stuff and quickly fled the scene.

Jake turned to the policeman. "Does your gun have real bullets in it?"

"It does, young fella. Guns are dangerous weapons, you know," the officer smiled.

"I know," Jake replied in a very serious voice. "My mommy won't let me have a real gun until I'm a grown up." He shook his head, "She won't even let me have a BB gun until I'm twelve." He sighed, "That's a long time."

"Well, when you're twelve you'll be right ready, I'll bet." He paused and turned to me, offering to show Jake the police cruiser if that would help.

Jake and the officer were barely out of the door when Lucy began to cry, burying her head in Mark's shoulder. Patting her back gently, he murmured, "There, there, baby, it'll be all right. I'll see you really soon. I promise."

I reached out to smooth Lucy's hair.

Lucy lifted her tear stained face and wailed, "I hate you! Don't touch me. I hate you, I hate you!" Then she broke down into wracking body sobs, hiding her face in Mark's chest.

Sliding past me, Mark carried the sobbing child down the hall and out the door.

Chapter 23

I wove through the winding streets on the way to the highway with Lucy in the back seat crying, and Jake solemnly silent in the seat beside me. Glancing frequently in the rearview mirror, I wondered when Lucy would stop and what I could say to her that would matter. Nothing came to me, so I drove in an eerie vacuum navigating continuous traffic and hoping I could really do this. More than once, I wondered if what I had done was the right thing. If it wasn't, I had screwed up all our lives even more and would be paying the price for years. And the final tally of my decisions might not even be counted until much later. I prayed for strength and a way to see this through, because I firmly believed it was the right thing to do. My life with Mark was over, and it was my job to take care of our children the best I could.

Not even Jake spoke as I finally reached the Turnpike exit and picked up speed heading west. At the first rest area, I pulled off the highway and offered the big treat of a Coke with the bathroom stop. Lucy wanted no part of any reconciliation and remained stubbornly in the car as Jake and I stretched our legs and got drinks, Jake asking me anxiously why Lucy was so sad. He was even willing to give her 'shotgun' if it would make her better. All I could do was hug him extra hard and reassure him Lucy would be all right.

Back in the car, I handed Lucy a cold Coke, her favorite. She just glared at me, shook her head and jerked away.

"Lu, I know you're upset but you'll see Daddy soon, and I want to be with you too."

She did not respond.

"Sweetie," I cajoled. "Memaw and Pop have missed you and so has Jamie and all your friends at school. And Jake, too." I reached over and ruffled his hair.

"You can sleep in my room when we get home. I have a new room in our new house!" Jake offered, taking a big gulp of the Coke.

"I don't want to sleep in your dirty old room in any house, and I hate that school!" Lucy snapped. Her eyes filled with tears and her face colored red with rage as she railed, "I want to go back to our real home with Daddy! I know that you just want to be with Sam, and I know that Daddy is sick and that you don't care if he dies cause then you could be with Sam. Daddy told me!"

Open mouthed, I gaped at my small daughter. The hurtful words and the venomous outpouring were more than I had ever anticipated. Undone by the day's drama and an overwhelming sense of failure, I laid my forehead on the steering wheel and broke down, my shoulders wracked with sobs.

Kneeling on his seat, Jake began to cry as he reached over and put his arms around me.

For a few moments, we sat that way, the sounds of sadness punctuated by the droning traffic noise at the busy rest stop. After a time, I lifted my tear stained face and kissed away the salty tears coursing down Jake's burnished cheeks, gently helping him back into his seat, securing him in. I looked back at Lucy, but her face was obscured, turned away towards the window. Completely emptied out, I had no words. I started the car and got back on the turnpike.

Just past Sturbridge, the car began to overheat as it had earlier that day on the Cape. The air conditioner had been on since leaving Boston and the temperature gage now hovered perilously near the end of the red zone. I knew we had to be close; their exit was just one more down, but I could not risk it, so I pulled off as the immediate exit loomed and cruised into the nearest gas station when the car began to smoke.

"Mommy, there's smoke. Look!" Jake shrieked, pointing to the front of the car. "It's gonna blow up!"

I ordered Jake to stay put, promising him the car was not going to blow up. My eyes lifted toward the heavens, I pleaded, 'Okay. I get it. What next, God? What life lesson do you have for me in this one?' I waited and took in a deep breath. No thunderclaps or lightning bolts followed, so I took another deep breath, glanced in the rear view mirror at what seemed to be a sleeping Lucy, then, I got out, walked around to the front of the car and raised the hood. Smoke billowed out.

"See, Mom, I told ya, it's gonna blow!" Jake's excited voice alerted as he, of course, jumped out of the car and dashed away from the smoke plumes.

I knew we must not be far from the Connecticut line. Surely, this place had a phone and maybe someone who knew what was wrong with the car. It was getting late, and Mike and Ruth expected us before dark. I left Lucy in the car, and Jake and I walked to the small convenience store near the gas pumps. It was locked up, but there was a pay phone out front. Digging in my bag, I found change and fed it into the slot. Nothing. No dial tone, silence. I was so weary and wanted to quit. Just give in. Lie down, hold my kids and sleep until this was all over, no matter how long it took. There was a comforting beauty to Rip van Winkle and all the sleep kissed damsels. Taking Jake's hand, I led him back to the car, unsure of what to do next. Lucy was stirring, and the smoke had ceased. Just as I was opening the car door, a truck lumbered in to the station. Mike was behind the wheel. Reality finally suspended, and I tumbled headfirst right through the looking glass. Overcome by exhaustion, lack of food and the events of this interminable day, I slumped over the car, sobs overtaking my spent body.

My feet propped up on the worn ottoman, I sipped a steaming cup of Chamomile tea, sweet with honey and liberally laced with whiskey; in the doctor's words, preferable to a sleeping pill. Embraced in the rolled arms of the old leather chair, I mulled over the unusual string of events. 'No such thing as coincidences,' had been the Casadega medium's prescient words.

When I stopped crying earlier at the car, I realized Mike was beside me, his experienced physician's arm cradling my shaking shoulders. Somehow, he had water in the truck and carefully filled the radiator. The temp gauge in the car went down immediately. He had coolant at the house and figured that was all I needed.

I asked him how he had found us.

"When you didn't show up, Ruth and I figured something was wrong." He shrugged, a quiet smile playing at the corner of his mouth, "Well, it had been wrong all day, but you were lost or something."

"But how'd you fix on the exit?"

"Well, this one's closest to the house by the back roads and there is a pay phone. When it works. I figured you'd see the phone and maybe stop."

As we pulled into the driveway, Ruth came out on the porch with Eric and Claire close to her heels. Even Lucy seemed to have given up her anger for the time being and quickly was caught up with all the attention, disappearing into the house with the big kids.

Ruth held me in a tight embrace, her brown eyes critically scanning my body. "You are mighty thin, girl! Need to fatten you up. I've made loads of food, stuff from the garden, and baked your favorite cookies. Glad Mike found you!"

Time and fashion trends had not affected Ruth; tan khaki shorts, a sleeveless T-shirt and Clarks. Clothing seemed just too much to fuss about. Her chestnut hair simply cut in a short bob, her fingernails stained with whatever she had been putting up or digging in that day.

We all inhaled an abundant dinner of fresh butter and sugar corn, tomatoes, cucumbers and grilled chicken, and when the children drifted off, I filled them in on the court scene and Lucy's behavior. Ruth listened while Mike asked pointed questions about Mark's health and about how I was holding up.

"You can only do so much, you know, then, your body shuts down. It's a good defense and you need to listen to it," Mike insisted across the table, taking a sip of wine.

"I know, I know." I tried to make light of my near collapse at the car. "It was just a really rough day, and I didn't count on Lucy being so terribly angry and hurt. That's what sent me over the edge, I think."

"Well, you appear to be better now. I imagine the lack of food combined with big time stress did you in. Are you taking any medication?"

"Not right now," I shook my head. "I took Xanax to sleep in the beginning, but stopped and seem to be all right without it."

Ruth leaned over and put her hand on mine. "Well, you need to rest tonight. My God, what an ordeal." She scooted her chair back from the table. "I'm going to clean up and you sit or go on up to bed. I'll bring you some tea with added sleep value."

"Thanks. I'd love some sleepy tea. I'll stay downstairs for a while."

"If you have trouble sleeping, let me know. A half a sleeping pill will do the trick," Mike offered.

"I think I'll sleep. Since I nearly collapsed at the car, I know I'm exhausted."

"Yep, stress like what you've had, plus low blood sugar will do it every time. You need to take care of yourself."

It was clear he wanted to say more, but he waited before continuing, "I know you know this, but sometimes we need reminders. Mark's not going to give up. Remember, we used to say that he'd be the one to get us all out of the prison by digging with a spoon." He leaned in and cautioned pointedly, "Things will probably get worse."

I looked over at him without speaking and nibbled my lower lip.

"You have to look after yourself too. Even if means taking an anti-depressant for a while," he reached over and covered my hand with his huge palm. "We're here and will do anything we can to help. All you have to do is let us know."

That night safe, nestled in soft flannel sheets, covered with the light down comforter, peaceful sleep came easily. The children had come in to give good night kisses and check on me to make certain all was well. Claire, at 11 had taken Lucy in, and Lucy basked in the attention of the older child. Eric, who was nine, allowed Jake to play with his Nintendo and sleep in the top bunk.

The morning sun filtered through the simple tab curtains. My eyes squinted open, the aroma of coffee and something baking wafted under the slightly ajar door. Offering a silent prayer of thanks, I got up, stretched and padded across the wide board pine floor to the window, pulling the curtain aside. Deep blue sky, dappled with cottony clouds, summer fragrances, and a light breeze, fluttered the curtain. No bad dreams, just a flirtation with calm. Smell the roses, Sam used to remind me.

The whoops of Jake declaring victory over whatever alien menace threatened his immediate game world jolted me out of my reverie. I grabbed the robe left conveniently on the door and headed downstairs.

"Morning," Ruth sang out when I entered the kitchen. "Coffee's over there, mugs in that cabinet over the pot and the blueberry muffins will be out in a flash." She turned from the sink where she was cutting cantaloupe, frowning at the miniscule melon, "I wish we could grow decent melons, but the season's just too short. Mike had early rounds at the hospital."

Pouring coffee, I took my cup and sat at the breakfast table which overlooked the lush flower garden that encircled the terrace. Cosmos, rudbekia and foxglove stood sentinel above the babies' breath and flowing nasturtiums.

"Your flowers look gorgeous. We can grow cantaloupe, but the heat kills the perennials. It's one thing I miss about New England, the summer flowers."

"But you can grow them in the winter can't you?" Ruth came and sat down across from me.

"Well, some of them," I took a sip of the hot coffee and smiled over at Ruth. "Thank you so much for being here and for all of this. I don't know what I would have done. I was pretty fried."

"I'm just happy I was home when you called. We're glad you thought of us, and for once," she grinned, "I'm glad we live across the state line."

I glanced up at the clock on the wall. "I want to drive as far as I can today. It's 8:00 and won't get dark until 9:00. Think I can do ten hours?"

"Are you nuts? You probably can, but the munchkins will kill each other. Figure on maybe seven hours at the most."

"That'll get me north of DC, right?"

"Yeah, stop where there is a pool, let them swim, have a good supper and get an early start the next day. Are you going to Jacksonville to your folks or all the way to Mt. Dora?"

I told her I wasn't sure, but did need to talk to my folks, realizing they would be worried, since I hadn't called. Bless them, they'd paid the considerable lawyer costs.

"Call now. Use the phone in Mike's office. The muffins are done."

When I came back into the kitchen, the muffins had been artfully arranged in a handmade basket. Cantaloupe slices alternated with ham and wedges of lime decorated a cobalt platter. Ruth was busily packing a small cooler with sandwiches, fruit, and cookies.

"You'll just need drinks. I don't have soda, and I know that's the easiest thing on a road trip."

I put my arm around her shoulders thanking her with a peck on her cheek.

She turned and hugged me back. "I wish we could do more. I'm so angry with Mark for what he did and how he's behaving now. I know he's suffering, but I am just not ready to make any kind of peace with him yet." She added, "What did your parents say?"

"Of course they fussed that I didn't call them yesterday, but when I told them the whole messy story they calmed down. They said to tell you all hello and thanks." I paused, "And they want me to come there before I go home. They'll follow me to Mt. Dora and our new place."

"That makes sense. It's not the time to be stoic and alone. With your friend, Sam far away, and the college group not all back, it'll be good to have them there."

"It will, I just hate to have them worry about all this. They're getting old."

"We'll worry about our kids until we die, like they do. Let them do what they can. Be glad you have them."

"You're right. I'll call them from the road once I know how far I've got to go and have them meet us at the rental house." The rental was two bedrooms with one bath and a small extra room, but it was cheap and in a great location. I had no idea what to expect. I'd left everything but clothes and basics in our home when I'd bolted, and reminded myself it was just stuff.

"The kids will be thrilled to have Memaw and Pop. Mom buys Cokes, Eskimo pies and every kind of potato chip they make. Dad watches cartoons with Jake and hoots at all the right moments," I smiled, picturing Dad and Jake glued to the television.

In the distance, I heard Lucy and Claire coming down the stairs. Jake was close behind, giggling about something.

All of a sudden, Lucy screeched, "Yuk, get that off me!"

Claire laughed as Jake shot into the kitchen, guilt written all over his face. "It's just silly putty, Mom."

Chapter 24

In comparison to the ordeal of Boston, the drive down to Florida seemed uneventful. Jake only threw up once and didn't torment a subdued Lucy, who listened to Care Bear tapes and said little. Our new place was like a doll house, but it was next door to the library, and we could ride bikes or walk to the quaint downtown and the pool. The routines of late summer and preparing for school were quickly established. First, I would drop Lucy and Jake at school. The church, where the kids had been in preschool had been all embracing of us and never did I worry about censure or fear. Jake would go home with his preschool teacher in the afternoons and then she'd get Lucy when she picked up her daughter who was a fifth grader. After work, I'd swoop by and pick both up, most times staying to visit. I felt so lucky, blessed even, that this had all worked and that the kids were taken care of and absorbed into this warm extended family. These were the folks who smiled and held Jake as he scooted under the kneelers at church, and had told Lucy how they liked her brother's Superman undies that she had insisted on wearing. Lu talked to Mark daily and seemed to have gotten past her anger over leaving Boston. His travels brought him to Florida fairly often and miraculously we'd worked out civil visits. He'd secured backstage passes when the group was in Orlando for our children and included the 'tweens' and any babysitters in our lives. Needless to say, this was a huge hit.

Sam wrote often. He was not coming back right away and planned on trying his luck at a non-profit in Boston for a while when he got back in the country. Disappointed, I understood. Since the college was beginning late, and in a way, starting over, this made sense. He had worked it out with Marsha, who was still the college president. There would be a job for him, but not until later in the year.

I devoured his letters.

'I miss you on a daily basis. You'd love it here. The water is clear all the way out and I've seen fish and yes, sharks that take my breath away. Don't worry, they're more shocked to see me.

The country is poor but unspoiled and the people hardworking and kind to each other and kind to strangers too. I've got more medical knowledge than anyone in the village, scary, right. The other day I treated a horrible burn on a guy. Wasn't sure if what I did was right, but the nearest hospital is a trek so it was me or nothing. Thank God, and I mean that! He's better. I'm just blown away by their courage and gratitude. Ate the other night with a family at their roadside stand. I'm not sure what we really ate, or even what they said, some of their speech patterns are unique, but the food was hot, delicious and cheap.

Give the rug rats a big hug and tell them to be good to their mom. I love you. I don't know what that means long term or where this will take us, but I know that the way I feel is a true thing that doesn't go away.'

Slowly, I ran my fingers over the smudged ink as if this act might conjure an elusive image, then folded the letter, put it back in the envelope and tucked it away with the others in the bedside table drawer. I never doubted Sam's love, it was the timing that continually challenged it all.

The holidays came and went without incident. Mark took the kids to Disney the day after Christmas, and I spent a quiet post-holiday with my parents in our small Mt. Dora house. Mom didn't even cook; we ate dinner at the hotel, surely, a first in my family. After they went back home, I got a call from Sam that he would be in Ft. Lauderdale with his family in January and could we find some time? His plans were to return to the college in late March after spring break. Enrollment for this mini-mester was low, and the 'real' semester wouldn't begin until month's end. I was elated and of course, I'd find time!

Annie was enlisted to take the kids. She would meet me half way to Jacksonville on the Friday of MLK weekend, and Sam and I would pick the kids back up on the following Monday afternoon. He was due to fly back to Boston from Ft. Lauderdale on Tuesday night, then pack up his meager belongings and drive down to Florida sometime in March.

After the long anticipated and intimate weekend, Sam and I pulled into the taco place where we were meeting Annie and the kids. We hung out in the car and waited. Annie was always punctual, so I began to be concerned after about a half hour. Using the pay phone in the restaurant, I called her house. No answer. Just as I was walking out, I saw the 'kid mobile' as we called her anemic small van, drive in. She stopped next to where I'd parked, and I saw only two heads, the boys; I assumed Lucy was asleep which was odd since she usually got to ride shotgun with her Aunt Annie. Stepping to the driver's side, I reached for the door. Annie was slumped over the steering wheel, and the boys were eerily quiet. I did not see Lucy. Sam had gotten out of the car and came to stand next to me. I heard Jake shout out for me to open the back door. Annie picked up her head, stared at me and opened the door, stumbling out of the van.

"I'm so sorry. I didn't know what to do. I called the police." She ran her hand through her short hair and then covered her mouth.

Sam moved to the back door and the boys hopped out.

"Dad came and Lucy went with him. He was in a big car with a big man." Jake offered, running and grabbing my hand.

Jamie put his arm around his mother.

"I honestly don't know how I even got here. I am so sorry." Annie looked at me, her eyes filling with tears.

I had said nothing during this short exchange of less than five minutes. Time had stopped, and it seemed like I had been witnessing a long scene in someone else's play.

Sam spoke first, addressing the boys, "Let's go inside and sit down, get a snack. I'll take the guys inside. Annie, are you okay with that?"

She said nothing.

I nodded to Sam as the boys ran ahead into the restaurant.

Annie reached for my hand. "I couldn't do anything. I tried. I tried to reason with Mark." She mumbled something and covered her face with her trembling hands. Taking her hands down, she bit hard on her bottom lip in a futile attempt to quell the tears. "He took her. I called the police!" Annie gulped for air. "Jake. Jake is here. He's okay."

She rocked back and forth, holding her hands around her arms, her shoulders shaking. "I'm so sorry. I couldn't do anything. The driver, the man who with Mark in the car, I think he had a gun. Oh God, I'm so sorry." Burying her head in my chest, her body heaving, she started to sob.

The quivering began in my hands and snaked down my body. I clutched Annie, holding on tight. The area around us seemed to be moving, and I was having trouble breathing, the steady low level traffic noise from the nearby road sounding like an airplane idling on the tarmac.

Annie lifted her tear stained face. "I called the police. They can't do anything because he's her father and so it's not kidnapping. I couldn't believe it, but they said there was really nothing they could do." With the back of her hand she swiped at the tears running down her cheek. "You need to call that lawyer. Maybe he can do something."

I managed to utter a feeble 'when did Mark show up'?

She continued in a manic rant, "Mark came about three or four hours ago. I made him coffee and tried to reason with him. You know like they tell you to do in those self-defense courses when you might be attacked. No one was home in the neighborhood when Mark got here. He planned that. He told me. He said he could have taken Lucy anytime he wanted to, but because it was me he didn't snatch her in the mall or at the skating rink, so I wouldn't freak out. I begged him not to do this to me, that the kids were on my watch. I'd been his friend. He said that was un- fucking fortunate. I'd made my choice as your friend."

She took a breath. "What a bastard! Then, he said he could have taken any of the kids, anytime. He's been watching for days, and kept up with where they were, when he talked to Lucy."

In a monotone, I asked her where he was heading. She didn't know, but Mark had told her not to bother calling the police because they wouldn't do anything.

Annie glanced around the car and spotted her purse. Her hand quivering, she took out her cigarettes, tapped one out, struck a match and took a long pull holding the smoke in. She slowly blew out the smoke. "I'm smoking in public. Lord, I never do that." She took another drag. "I don't care. I must be in shock or something. Anyhow, Mark had this huge body guard man with him. Like the goon squad. When I told Lucy to come with me and reached out for her, Mark told me to step aside. The guy opened his jacket and touched whatever he had in a holster." She paused, "Then Mark told me to get out of the way and for Lucy to get in the car."

"Where were the boys?" I gripped on to the car for support.

"Right there. It was horrible! Jake said he wanted to go too and Mark told him," she hesitated, her voice breaking, "Mark told him, he told him no, he just wanted Lucy." Annie's eyes filled up as she tapped the lingering ash from her cigarette. "He's really crazy, Kathy."

"Oh dear, God." I collapsed over the car and covered my head with my arms.

Gently, Annie put her arms around my waist and led us toward the restaurant where Sam and the boys were waiting.

Anyhow," Annie paused, before we went in, "for what it's worth, Jake seems okay. He didn't really understand or even really hear and that's good. The boys are so young and they forget and go on. The guy and the gun scared us all. Even Lucy seemed worried."

I gazed back at her vacantly, realizing I needed to call my attorney, but I didn't know his number. It was at home.

Annie looked over at me and saw the glazed stare in my eyes. "Honey, we'll get her back." She put her hand on my shoulder. "Mark is a sick, crazy man but he won't hurt Lucy. He loves her in his demented way. She'll be all right."

Chapter 25

My tongue danced around my parched lips. Gritty particles of silt made it hard to swallow and my eyes watered, burning, remnants of the sand storm gathered like gnats in the corners. I wanted to wipe my eyes, but I couldn't seem to manage, only one hand worked; the other was pinned tight, caught beneath a wagon wheel. Somehow, I knew that I had to move. Night would come soon and the jackals would be out, feeding on the weak.

In the distance, a muted voice was urging me awake. Faint at first, the voice got louder, and then a small hand caressed my cheek.

"Mommy, Mommy, don't cry anymore, I'm here," Jake mumbled and snuggled in, turning over on my sleep paralyzed, outstretched arm.

I opened my eyes to the little boy's face and cautiously wiggled the fingers on the useless arm. I kissed him on the head. "I'm not really crying, those are just sleep tears. Move over for a minute, baby, my arm's asleep."

"How does your arm sleep?" he questioned, a puzzled look on his face.

"Oh, sometimes the blood doesn't get to it and circulate and it gets numb."

"Oh," he said, "wake up arm." He jiggled my hand and spoke directly to the lifeless arm.

Lifting my arm, I smiled, "You are amazing! Look it's moving."

"I am Jake the Magician, da dah," he waved his hand, wand - like over my body.

My nose in his tousled hair, I breathed in that child sleep smell and grabbed him in a fierce hug, holding him tight. Silently, I thanked the Lord that he was here and that Lucy was all right. As if he could read my mind, he turned up his small face and asked me when would Lucy come back? I took his hand and told him honestly that I didn't know.

Mark was healthy for now, but the disease was insidious and would rear its head at some point. I hoped she'd be back before that happened. Surely, he would see that.

Jake said nothing for a moment as he scrutinized my face, looking intently at me with his dad's eyes. "Can I call her?"

I paused, trying to keep up a brave front telling him that Daddy had a new number and when he called back we'd have it. My lawyer had said there wasn't much to do immediately but wait. He was certain Mark would be in touch again. He had called once, on the Tuesday morning after Sam had gone.

I had spoken to my parents earlier and Sam had talked with Marsha. My folks, thankfully, hadn't paid attention to my telling them we were okay and arrived shortly after I'd gotten off the phone with Mark. His one way conversation had washed over me like a tidal wave, tumbling over and over, and I couldn't get to my feet to take a breath. Mostly, I remember his solemn promise that if I persisted in pursuing anything legal, he would hide Lucy somewhere, and I'd never see her. His position with the rock group afforded him privacy, protection, and insulation from fans and any others without clearance.

My parents had taken a quick look at the situation and fed me a leftover Xanax, insisting I take a short nap. Flattened by grief, I floated in and out with people talking over my head. There were lots of voices. If I stayed under I couldn't hear them. I could hold my breath and stay put. There I was safe. I think by the time I was able to get out of bed a day or two had passed.

While I had been missing, Mark's Dad had called. Apparently, the conversation had been troublesome for all. In my parents' retelling it went something like this.

My mom handing the phone to my dad, "I just can't. You'll have to talk to him."

My dad, gentlemanly, was direct, but brief. "I realize there are always two sides to any story, Jack, he's your son, and he's ill, but he's gone over the edge and you know it. He has our granddaughter, and God willing he'll take care of her. You're a couple of hours away and can't help if there's trouble."

Mom said she hadn't seen Daddy so angry since a neighbor kid plowed down his silver maple tree doing wheelies on his motorcycle.

"Well, I'm pleased Lucy is doing fine and likes the school."

Mom said Dad was rigid, his mouth set in a thin line. "Yep, I realize he's her father and he loves her, but he's not quite sane, not at this point. Not physically well either, remember."

"Yes, well, we'll be here for a while to help out. Goodbye." Then, he put down the phone, looked around the room, spotted his pipe and marched out to the porch where he sat puffing away, as if the smoke exorcized demons.

Eventually, after about a week, I forced myself to emerge from my mental cocoon, a bit thinner and pale. Thankfully, colleagues had covered at work and my parents had settled in.

Late one afternoon, I wandered into the galley kitchen where my mom was fixing supper. Surprised, she looked up from the counter.

I put my arms around her waist and rested my head on her shoulder.

She turned around and hugged me close, asking me hopefully, if I was hungry. She'd made macaroni and cheese, and okra and tomatoes, two of my (and Lucy's) favorites.

I leaned in to my mother's comfortable chest and breathed deeply, taking in the familiar fragrances, Estee Lauder and Ivory soap.

That night, the four of us sat down at the small table and Jake wanted to say the blessing. Squeezing his eyes tightly shut, his hands folded, he began, "Dear God, thank you that Mommy's not sick anymore and bless Lucy and Daddy and our whole family and thank you for the macaroni." He peeped out from under his heavily fringed lashes at the grownups. "And make Lucy come home soon. Amen."

My folks stayed on for another week. I went back to work, the days following their normal routine, minus Lucy, who called almost daily to chat and assure us she was doing fine. Soon she and Daddy were traveling across country all the way to California with the band and she was so excited. It was okay that she was missing school because the trip would be educational, the principal had agreed with Daddy.

Jake always talked with Mark, but most of his conversation consisted of when were Daddy and Lucy coming home. Mark's answer that they'd see him soon seemed to pacify Jake for a while, until Lucy called again.

The next week in David's therapy office, I glanced down at my hands. "So, that's about it, I guess. I had a major meltdown. Thank God for my folks, all of y'all and," I paused, "I'll be okay."

David smiled his soft smile and waited to see if I had more to say. When I said nothing, he began, "You'll be all right. It'll take a while and the medication will help."

David, observing my expression, held up his hand in a stop gesture. "I know, I know what you think about meds, but bear with me. You must sleep or you'll be of no use to anyone, Jake or yourself included. The medication is a low dose and will take the edge off. You probably won't dream much either."

I raised my eyebrows. "Well, that would be a good thing. The dreams have gotten terrible. I had the pinned beneath the wheel one again the other night."

"Your dreams are pretty powerful. It's how your mind processes all this, which can be a good thing, but you need to sleep too. And, the meds may not stop them all together, but they'll help." He continued, "So how are you today?"

"Oh, I'm all right, I guess. I still can't believe that Mark took Lucy." My voice dropped as I went on, overcome with sadness. "And that she wanted to be with him so much..." my voice trailed off.

"But you know that Mark manipulated her. She's just a child and he laid his well- being on her. Remember in her note to you she wrote that Daddy needs me. That's totally screwed up. Parents don't rely on kids. It's the other way around."

"I know," I tried to squash the building tears. "I miss her so much. And Jake," I waited, "not a day goes by that he doesn't ask when she's coming home." My eyes filled. "Why do you think that Jake's never mentioned Mark saying he didn't want him?"

David's gaze wandered to the window. He waited for a moment before responding. "He's young, he's got you, his anchor, and it probably didn't register with him the way it would have with an older child."

"Do you think he might later on, you know, it's all repressed and will surface in some bizarre behavior when he's ten?"

"It's hard to say. You know more about child development than I do. Psychologically, I think Jake is quite resilient and has you as his constant. Lucy is the one to be more concerned about. Even though she's the "desired" child by her dad, the burden Mark has placed on her is enormous. Imagine feeling responsible for taking care of a parent at her age."

He shook his head, a frown worrying his brow. "Kids who become caretakers have a long journey to healing. The longer they are in that role the longer it takes to come back to childhood."

The welled up tears overflowed, and I swiped at my eyes with the back of my hand.

David handed me a tissue.

I didn't know I was capable of the immense anger that suddenly engulfed me. I looked hard at David and whispered, "I think I would have killed him you know, if the kids were sick."

David sat quietly, saying nothing.

"I thought about it over all those months of not knowing. If I was dying and had to watch my children die, I couldn't have endured it and not done anything once I knew the truth."

I shifted my eyes back to David. "It's sort of a scary thing to know that about yourself."

"Well, you can still kill him, symbolically. Probably, a better choice." He smiled, the corners of his mouth turned up slightly. "It's a good way to deal with some of the rage."

"Will it help?"

"It won't hurt."

"I'll feel silly.

"And so, your point?"

"What do I do?"

"Close your eyes and imagine Mark sitting over there," he gestured to the empty chair by the window. "Use the breathing techniques we've talked about. Now, when you visualize him in your mind sitting in the chair, use your hand as a gun. Open your eyes and squeeze the trigger as many times as you want to. Scream at him, tell him what you'd want to say to him while you pull the trigger."

I shut my eyes and began to breathe, concentrating on the rising and falling of my diaphragm. I felt myself slowing down and focusing inward as my breathing became more rhythmic. Slowly, I raised my hand, my arm extended, index finger straight out, thumb poised in position. Opening my eyes, I aimed at the empty chair where I'd placed Mark.

Crouching forward in the chair, I leveled my arm and began the imaginary volley of shots. I screamed every obscenity I knew, yelled that I despised him for what he'd done, and he could go rot in hell!

I finally stopped and dropped my arm, slumped back in the chair, sweat beading on my lip. Frozen, I stared into space.

"What do you feel right now?"

"Sad and an overwhelming sense of loss."

"What's going on with your body?"

"Oh," I glared at him through misted eyes, "that. Did I tell you how much I hate this Gestalt stuff you do?"

"Many times."

"Well. So, my breathing is slowing down, and the tightness is leaving my back. And I'm not sweating anymore." I put my palms to my cheeks. "My face is really hot and my throat still feels tight. The back of my neck is getting looser." I wiped my nose with the crumpled tissue as the tears started down my hot cheeks.

"Keep going."

"I don't know how else I feel other than I'm crying AGAIN! And I still hate him. That hasn't gone away."

"I didn't expect it would."

"What good was it then?"

"It's out, that's it. Simple. And you've felt what it's like to let go."

He waited for me to take in what he said. "You know we've had a number of discussions that you live in your head. It's where you are most comfortable. What you just experienced isn't your head. It's your gut. It's where you feel, not think. It's different for you, it's out of your comfort zone." He smiled and stood up. "You did well. Think about the meds. They're not evil, a crutch for the weak. Taking them for a short while may help."

Chapter 26

We had spoken to Lucy mid-week. They were in California and all was well, so I looked forward to a quiet weekend with Jake, when early Saturday morning the telephone rang. On my first cup of coffee, I ignored the phone and decided to let the answering machine get it. Barefoot in my short gown, I stopped on the way out of the room when I heard the clipped New England emanating from the message tape.

"I was hoping to find you in." Mark's dad paused with an audible sigh, "Well, it's Saturday morning and you and Jake must have gotten out early. Call me as soon as you get in. It's important."

On Wednesday, when Lucy had called, she'd been bursting with excitement. They were on their way north to San Francisco and had been in Los Angeles at an awards ceremony where she and Daddy sat at the table with Elton John. Not only that, she reported breathlessly, but she was in the music video that the group had recently made.

Jake wanted to know who was Elton John? And, did she see the Ninja Turtles and did she know he was going to the Nickelodeon show with Jamie? (Everything is relative after all.)

That was the last time Lucy had called, and I figured we'd talk to her today or tomorrow.

Before I started the day, I might as well find out what Jack wanted. He picked up on the first ring.

"Hi, I just got your message."

"Thank goodness you called," Jack responded, his typical reserved tone different. "Listen, I can't find Mark and I'm worried."

Puzzled, I asked him what he meant, that he couldn't find Mark. He and Lucy were in California.

He went on as if I were truly simple, he knew that. What he meant was that Mark's not at the hotel where he's supposed to be.

Pausing to be to be certain of the day, I told him I spoke with Lucy on Wednesday, and they were leaving LA and taking the tour bus or driving a rental up the coast to San Francisco. They were staying at the Fairmont.

"Yes, I know that, too," Jack answered, emphatic. "What I'm telling you is that he's not there."

"That's crazy. There must be some mistake. Whom did you speak to?"

"I'm not mistaken," he reiterated, an edge of panic creeping into his voice. "You probably didn't know, but he was sick in Los Angeles and running a high fever. You know how stubborn he can be. I pleaded with him to go to the doctor there, but he wouldn't listen to me, said he had run fevers before. I even called Phillip and begged him to talk some sense into Mark. He promised he would try but wasn't hopeful; they've never been close like some brothers are, even as kids."

"Did you tell the hotel it was an emergency and you were his father?"

"Of course. I did all that. No one can get through to the group unless they have a certain level of clearance. Mark didn't give me any."

"What? Why not?"

"I don't know. You know how he is."

I drew in a deep breath, and told him to give me the number of the hotel. I'd call and see what I could find out. There had to be some reasonable explanation. I assumed he and Lucy were there and it was a registration error.

"Call me as soon as you know something. I'm afraid he's really sick this time." He hesitated, "And if he is, really sick, who is taking care of Lucy?"

I refused to let Jack's fretfulness make me worry. Mark would make sure that Lucy was cared for. There was probably just a mix up with names.

The concierge at the Fairmont assured me in his unctuous voice that Mr. Hayes had not checked in and that no, it was simply impossible to be connected to the manager of the rock group. My name was not on the list of those cleared to be put through and yes, madam, blah, blah, blah, the group was staying in his hotel, and he was in charge so he would know.

I wracked my brain trying to remember where Mark and Lucy had stayed in Los Angeles and rummaged through the trash can hunting for the number that Lucy had given me when we last spoke. Not finding the paper, but recalling the hotel, I called directory assistance and got the number. The desk answered on the first ring and assured me Mr. Hayes was not there. All the entourage had checked out.

Overwhelmed with frustration, I refused to let rising anxiety escalate, assuring him this was an emergency and was he certain?

"Yes, madam, (this must be the moniker for snotty west coast hotels; frankly, I preferred ma'am) I'm sure he's not here."

There had to be some reasonable explanation for this. I delayed calling Jack back because he feared the worst. Mark was sick somewhere and Lucy was with him. Why Lucy hadn't called me was what I didn't understand as my mind began to run rampant and race through the horrors of a child lost, alone with sick parent, stuck on the road and no telephone in sight, terrified.

My bare feet slapped on the cold floor and I shivered, trying to quell the gnawing anxiety that was slowly growing, taking over like a malignant Pac-Man in one of Jake's games. So long as I didn't give voice to the fears they wouldn't be real. When I was a little girl, I thought if you didn't talk about scary dreams they wouldn't come true, the same for wishes; don't tell when you blow out the birthday candles or you won't get your wish.

The day passed and no word from Mark or Lucy. Jack had not heard either. I wracked my brain as to the next step. My Boston friend, Kate, was an attorney in San Francisco, and I knew she'd done free legal work for people with AIDS. If Mark was in the hospital, she might know which ones were more likely to serve people with AIDS. I was debating about calling her when the phone rang. Hopeful that it was Lucy, I grabbed for the phone.

"Hello, don't hang up, I'm here."

"Hi, I'm glad you're there," Sam said. "I was gonna leave a suggestive message, hoping you'd hear it sometime before you said goodnight."

I was so glad to hear his voice and unloaded before he said anything more.

"Lucy and Mark are missing, Jake knows something is wrong and has been glued to me all day, and I'm grimly waiting for an asteroid to hit the house as we speak."

"Well, not to downplay your cosmic fear theory, but first you said Lucy and Mark are missing. What do you mean?"

I filled him in on the details of the day.

"Can't you get through to someone in the group who should know?"

"You'd think so, but Mark didn't put me or his dad on his call through list. It's like getting through to the President. I think he's sick and that he's in the hospital, somewhere. The problem is he could be anywhere between LA and San Francisco." I waited, inhaled deeply to clear my head and continued, "And Lucy may not be with him."

"Yeah, well, she may not be. She's probably fine and with the group in the Fairmont, but he'll know where she is."

As I prattled on as if Sam hadn't said a word, I realized how worried I was. "Oh, she must be so frightened. She hasn't called, so she must not be able to. If she was with him in the hospital wouldn't the doctor or nurses try to find me?"

"Yes, if Mark wasn't cogent, but if he's talking and seems to be okay they'd probably stay out of it. I don't think she's with him. He'd have gotten someone from the crew to get Lucy and take care of her. As self-centered as he is, he takes care of her physically at least."

I waited a moment to respond, then told him about my lawyer friend, whom I'd decided to call. Once I knew where Lucy was I would find a way to bring her home.

Later that afternoon, I called Kate and filled her in. We'd been friends and colleagues since our twenties, and she also knew Mark. Eager to help, she would let me know once she found him. And she wanted the name of his Boston attorney.

Exhausted from the day, I tucked Jake in and fell asleep quickly. About midnight, Kate called announcing she had found them both.

"Oh, thank God, and thank you. Where are they?"

"Mark is here in the hospital, like we figured, and Lucy is fine. Mark told me where to find her. She's at the Fairmont with the wardrobe matron, an older Hispanic woman who barely speaks English, which is why Lucy couldn't call. I had Mark call her, and I'm here at the hotel now. Hold on, Miss Lucy's eager to talk."

I struggled to keep my voice under control as Lucy's childlike sounds chirped through the phone filling me on all the details of why she hadn't called. Basically, it had been like I figured, Mark had gotten sick and the 'group' had taken charge. Thank the good Lord and all of them!

Kate came back on the line after sending Lucy and the helper out for a Coke.

"It wasn't that difficult. There are only so many hospitals who have AIDS patients and I know them all. I just made a few calls."

"And you found him?"

"I did. After a totally, inappropriate conversation with his lawyer."

It turned out that she had done some cross country legal work with the Boston woman and called her to find out what she knew, which of course is not kosher, given attorney client privilege. In the process, Kate had unloaded on her that her very ill client was not the poor maligned victim she probably believed him to be. Kate thought she'd be lucky if the woman didn't file a complaint, but as she eloquently remarked, 'fuck it,' I found Lucy and told Mark what I thought of his behavior!

She then gave me her take on Mark's health. "He's really sick and they're pumping him full of every anti-viral thing they've got. It's just one opportunistic infection after the other, which is typical with AIDS folks. Apparently, he's better than he was when he came in. He'll probably be ready to leave in a few days if he doesn't contract something else. This won't kill him. The god awful disease isn't finished with him yet." She stopped to take a breath, "I've seen guys go on for months. One of my close friends lasted for over a year like this. Usually pneumonia gets you in the end."

I felt my throat close as the old panic rose, remembering the white hot fear I had lived with, the terror that had lurked for me and the kids. Not able to utter a word, I barely breathed in an effort to suppress the rising tremors. As angry as I was with Mark's deception, no one deserved to die for having sex. No one deserved this. This disease played with you, like a cat and an injured mouse. It was a slow torture and then, a miserable death that you can't escape unless you beat it to the punch. You know, do yourself in.

"Kath, you still there?" Kate asked and then continued, not expecting a response. "I'm sorry to be so blunt about his health and all, but you need to know the facts. He looks awful, and I don't think he's got long, and there is no way in hell that he can take care of Lucy. Every time he gets sick with something he gets weaker. And he knows it." She stopped, waited for a comment from me and when I said nothing, continued. "You know how we always said he'd dig us out of a landslide with a spoon if we needed him, well, that's what keeps him going. That, and the kids." She sighed. "He really does love his kids." She stopped talking. "Listen, they're coming back. I gotta regroup. Who's coming to get Lucy?"

Outside the smudged airport window, I marveled at how the cottony clouds beckoned; they appeared so close, scattered in the bright blue, solid, almost welcoming, yet, they were ephemeral, just gases, fleeting, they shifted in an eye blink. So much had changed from the last time I waited in this airport, standing still, regarding the clouds. The past couple of years seemed like a page from someone else's tabloid life story, but this was real, all mine and I was tethered to the earth for now and grateful for every moment I had to watch the clouds.

I thought about Hazel, the Casadega medium, her sense of prescience. There was something to be said for her predictions about ancestors protecting me (this was long before the theory of genetic immunity) because here I still was, perched on the precipice, not knowing what was ahead or where the journey would lead.

A turning point had occurred for me that day in David's office, when I symbolically shot Mark. Maybe it was that enough time had passed; maybe it was the acceptance that the children and I were truly all right; maybe it was just the awareness that life and time on earth are precious and not to be wasted on anger.

Closing my eyes, the familiar words worked their way into my consciousness. "Forgive us our trespasses as we forgive those who trespass against us." Perhaps, that was the strength that would allow for peace and the forgiveness to move on.

Mark's brother, Dick had volunteered to go to California to get Lucy. He wanted to see Mark and didn't mind the trip. We'd exchange Lucy in the airport and then he was back to Boston. When he called from Mark's room to update me, the visceral dread I now associated with hospitals and AIDS patients crept in: the medicinal smells that caused the bile to build in my throat while I swallowed back the rancid acid; the hurried hustling of weary staff averting their eyes as they passed; red signs posted on closed doors, use caution when entering, contagious disease alert; no visitors but family allowed. Nurses masked, gowned and gloved emerged silently from the sterile rooms. No flowers, balloons or well- wishers who waited anxiously for news of a successful surgery, a miraculous recovery or the platitude frequently proffered, that with time this too will heal.

When Dick arrived at the hospital, Mark was lying motionless on the bed attached to a multitude of tubes, one in his nose, one in a port in his chest, and one stuck at an uncomfortable angle in his frail blue veined hand. His skin pallid, the color of cold grits, his brother had tried hard not to stare at this shrunken shell, the man who had once been so handsomely powerful.

Lucy and Uncle Dick walked hand in hand off the plane, and when Lucy rushed into my arms it was hard for me not to cry. She seemed relieved. Ever thankful to Dick, I hugged his neck and reminded him to let me know when he was safely home.

As we pulled into the driveway of our tiny rental, Jake flew out the back door. Lucy jumped out of the car and into Jake's small arms, laughing as he shrieked at her. No pouty face, no sad words, just apparent joy to see her rambunctious brother (by dark they'd probably be fussing).

"I've been sleeping in your bed every night and sometimes Mom even lets me have Fat Ivan (the cat) there too. Maybe, she'll let you have him stay with you. I can still stay if you're scared or you can sleep in my room. And we have real homemade cookies, the kind you like with the raisins and real Cokes, *real* Cokes," he emphasized, reverence in his voice, "cause Memaw and Pop are here, and Memaw said she'll make macaroni too."

He stopped to take a breath, glanced over at me as I stood nearby. "Mommy, she's back!" Coming over to me, he grabbed my hand and kissed it, then asked if Daddy was coming back too.

Hesitating and before I could respond, Lucy answered back, matter of fact, "Daddy is sick for now, but I talked to him and he said he'd be better and then, he'll come see us."

Just then, the door opened and Mom and Dad stepped out. Seeing them, Lucy bolted and flew into Dad's outstretched arms, "Poppy!" she yelled as he bent down and lifted her up. Mom leaned over and began smothering Lucy with kisses, the tears glistening in her crinkled eyes, "Oh, darling baby, we missed you so much."

Chapter 27

The last time we saw Mark was around Thanksgiving. He was in Florida with the now rock star group and came to see the children. Skeletal thin, his skin ashy and splotched with the tell-tale red sarcomas that many AIDS patients had, his once strong, deep voice weakened by the treatments and damaged by the earlier radiation. The pain and sadness I felt for him was palpable. That night, he slept in the lower bunk in Jake's room and fearful of the wheezing noises his dad made, Jake crawled into bed with me.

Earlier that day, I'd tried to make peace with Mark, offering him a place to stay as long as he needed it. He would have none of it, but something compelled me to keep going. When determined, I'd never been good at keeping my mouth shut.

"I don't care if you want to listen to me, but I'm going to say what I need to say to you. And somewhere deep in that part that you keep all yours, you will hear me and it will be remembered."

I stopped, shocked at the intensity and passion I had for what I was about to say. "I have loved you. I am the mother of your children and will always be, just like you will always be their father, even when you are gone. I find it hard to believe that you hate me, because I've done nothing but survive."

I took a breath and barreled on. "Hating is a waste of whatever precious energy you have left. I don't hate you anymore for what you did. I can't forgive you yet, but I pray that will come with time."

Slowly, as if the effort pained him, Mark finally spoke, telling me that I left him for another man and took his children away from him and that he would never have done that to me. But, he continued, even with all that, he loved me, never hated me and always wanted me back.

My eyes flooded with tears. After all this time, he would never believe that I didn't leave him for another man or because he had AIDS.

"It wasn't enough, what we had, the kids, us. I'd always wanted more than you could give me. And you knew my history. You knew I'd slept around, men and women. It was just sex, another thing to do. Another rush, an impulse. I couldn't help it. I got bored and had been for a while. You weren't part of that. I didn't even really consider you in the equation."

I stared at Mark, finding it hard to comprehend what I had just heard and involuntarily flinched, my eyes giving away feelings of disbelief at what he had shared. It seemed that David had been right. Mark's behavior was dictated by what he wanted and needed. Others didn't figure into the mix at all, really.

Mark saw my eyes reflect my thoughts, and continued, "You never were a good card player. You give it all away with those eyes." He sighed, "You are an attractive woman and smart too. That always kept me hooked. A little up tight in bed, but I really did love you. And, I am sorry and tried to make it up to you, but you took the kids and left me."

I couldn't say a word, stunned by what I had just heard. The tears that had begun to fall had stopped and dried in salty furrows on my cheeks. The next morning, Mark drove away.

The call came in the wee hours of grey dawn, the first blush of the Florida sun painting the horizon a watercolor wash of bridesmaid pink. Just light, the telephone's shrill jangling heard throughout the house, I grabbed the phone, mumbling a sleep, saturated hello.

It was Mark's father, Jack, his usual steely voice soft, choked. I clutched the phone with two hands as if it had a mind of its own and would make its way back to the safety of its cradle on the bedside table if I let go.

"It was this morning about a half hour ago. The nurse woke me. I'd dozed off I guess. We knew it wouldn't be long once the morphine drip started, but it happened so fast, in the end. He just stopped breathing. Thank God, it was peaceful, he'd been in such pain. But now it's over. He's gone."

"Oh, Jack, I'm sorry. I don't know what to say other than I'm so sorry. He's your son."

"I wasn't a good father, you know. I loved him and always gave in to him, and I didn't do that with the others. They resented that you know."

"Oh, you can never love your children too much."

Silence lingered. Then, "Well, so far," Jack continued, his stoic Irish shutting down further discussion. "I haven't called anyone else yet, but the coroner is on the way and the ambulance. The home health people knew what to do. The ambulance will take him to Rhode Island, to a funeral home there."

When I questioned why Rhode Island, Jack told me that funeral homes were particular about AIDS deaths. The nurses had warned him, so when Mark got worse, Jack had made some calls and the closest place that would take Mark was in Rhode Island. And this was 1992, outside liberal Boston.

"That's the way it is. He wanted to be cremated so they'll do it there and then someone will have to go pick up his ashes." He stopped talking, the mention of ashes alluding to the finality of Mark.

He asked when the kids and I might get up there, and I told him I'd make arrangements and try to fly out tomorrow.

"That'll be fine, there's nothing you can do here," He drew in a deep breath as though thinking through the propriety of death. "Just let me know once you get the flight times, and I'll have someone meet you. You don't need a car, Mark's is just sitting here."

"Okay, I'll call and let you know once I get times." Swallowing back the familiar lump, the years of emotional distance evaporating, I offered to come today if it would help him in any way. "Jack are you all right? I mean I know that's a dumb question, what I mean is you've been there all along with him and now that Libby (Mark's mother had died earlier that year) is gone and well, you don't need to be alone."

"I don't mind alone," the old Irishman responded. "I'm just thankful that he's not here the way he was. The other day I was changing his diapers, and I remembered when he was a baby. I never imagined I'd be doing it again when he was dying." He continued in a rush, "You know when he threw me out in January, I told myself that I'd stay gone. I'd had it. He made me so mad with that obstinate, arrogant way of his. But I came back. He's my son," he finished, trailing off as the muffled tears took over, the façade of constraint gone.

My words were punctuated by my own crying. "I can't imagine what it was like for you. He was my husband, the father of our children, and I believe that he did love us in his way. I can't believe that what we had for all that time was just a sham."

"Oh, he loved those children, he really did. Talking to them, even when he didn't have the breath to talk for long was all he lived for in the end."

I wiped the tears off my cheeks with the edge of the sheet as Jack outlined his plans for letting other family members know.

Then, he added, "I'm calling the priest to see about a funeral mass. It turns out that Mark met with him a few times."

"He met with the priest?"

"Yes, I found out because I ran into one of the women who worked in the parish office, and she asked how he was doing. Seems they'd been bringing him meals. It's strange isn't it that he did that, went to the priest, he was always so down on the church."

"He was. A severely lapsed Catholic as he put it. I'm glad he did that. Maybe it gave him some peace."

"I hope so," he replied. "Anyway, I'll talk to you later today once you know when you can get a flight."

I hung up the phone and sat staring out the window at the now golden day, my knees pulled up to my chin, adjusting the covers. The room was cold. This scene had been rehearsed in my head so many times. Each time Mark spoke to the kids, he was in a weakened state. They'd seen him that last time, his skin sallow, his lips bluish, caked with sores; his thin body wracked with a wheezing cough that doubled him over when he tried to talk for long. Even his amazing blue eyes had lost their luster. Jake had wanted to know how Daddy could breathe like that. Lucy told Jake to hush up, Daddy was sick. That was about four months ago and now Mark was gone.

My eyes wandered to the worn place in the Oriental rug that always scrunched up. I'd been determined to keep the rug even though I knew how threadbare it looked. Mark had disliked the rug, said I'd been taken by the "flaming" rug dealer. We'd argued, and I told him it was my money, and he had no taste. He smirked and replied that the guy saw me coming and knew I was an easy mark. Angry, I'd turned to storm out of our first apartment when he caught me by the hand, pulled me close and whispered that the rug might be good for something, as we tumbled to the hard floor and made love on the scratchy Oriental. The rug burns on my backside had lasted for days.

Sitting still on the bed for a few moments, the tears quietly falling, my mind played over other scenes, when we'd been happy. Finally, I got up, splashed water on my face and walked down the hall and into the kitchen. Getting out the coffee, I measured the water and soon the reassuring aroma permeated the room as the coffee made its familiar perking sound.

I glanced at the clock on the wall. Less than an hour had passed and a life had vanished. Where had he gone? His useless, shrunken body was empty, abandoned and soon would lie on a cold slab. His soul, whatever that is, was somewhere out there. I remembered the medium and her fear for Mark's mortal soul. My lips moving in a silent prayer for him, I prayed that he had made his peace and found rest. Somehow, I think he had.

The coffee stopped and I poured it into a cup, the hot steam misted my face as I breathed in the comforting smell and gripped the warm cup around my cold hands. A high pitched mewling pierced the quiet. Opening the door, kitty Fat Ivan dashed in, yowling and caressing my bare legs. The air outside felt chilly for March, the kids would need jackets. They should go in to school for a few hours, no reason to keep them home and I needed to call Marsha (and Sam). We'd need coverage for my classes. I reached out to shut the door and noticed one yellow daffodil had burst open in the Florida spring revealing its vanilla, petaled face. Yesterday, it had been tightly closed. The door ajar with the dappled sun on my face, I studied the perfect flower that had emerged from the gnarled, humble bulb I had planted deep in the warm ground last year. It was hard to believe it had been a whole year. After all this time, Mark's life was finally over.

Chapter 28

Jake fidgeted and wiggled on the hard wooden pew while I repeatedly shushed him as he asked one question after the other. I wondered why I cared what people thought about how the children behaved. None of us would be back in this church, and most likely, never see some of these folks again. A handful of Mark's friends and the cousin, who was like a sister to him, hadn't spoken nor acknowledged me. Here we were, bound together in mourning a life lost and people apparently were still judging me for not staying with Mark. Or maybe, they never liked me and now, didn't have to pretend.

A couple of the teenage stars and some of the production team had sneaked in quietly and settled in the back of the church attempting not to attract attention, (which was made difficult by the fur coat and designer shades sported by one of them). When the service ended, they hurried over to hug Lucy and Jake before making a quick getaway. Recognized by some of the young set at the funeral, they kindly gave autographs. I puzzled at what message their signatures on a funeral mass card might convey.

When sharing goodbyes with the friends who had come, my voice broke as I told them how much I appreciated the gesture. I'd assured my parents and the Florida group that they didn't need to attend the funeral. We'd need their help on the other end when we returned home.

Only the family was going to the cemetery. Mark had wanted his ashes buried at the cemetery on the Cape beside his mother's grave. Driving across the Sagamore Bridge, the children were quiet and somber. I grasped their small, mittened hands tightly and glanced over at Lucy who had not said a word since getting in the car. I reached out and put my arm around her shoulder and pulled her close.

She turned her face from the window and looked earnestly at me. "Do we really go to heaven when we die, Mommy?"

I stared at my serious and 'old beyond her years' daughter, "I believe we do."

"Is Daddy there now?"

"Is Grandma Libby there with Daddy?" Jake chimed in.

A soft smile played around my lips, as I told him I bet she was glad to see her youngest son.

The large car slid into the reserved space and we got out, bracing against the cold wind that blew across the water, while the frigid air whistled over the hill top and rustled the bare limbs of the naked trees. Elton John's poignant, 'Don't let the sun go down...' wafted out of a boom box. Mark had asked one of the nieces to be sure it was played. The only other sound was the muffled crying of the cousin/sister, her head bowed, her gloved hand gripping her husband's, her children standing silently.

The family gathered around the plot where a small hole had been made to hold the urn of ashes. Jack, eyes red rimmed and tired, clasped the container of ashes to his chest and turned to Lucy and Jake asking them to help him put this in the ground.

Obediently, Jake walked over to his grandfather. Lucy stood still, biting her lip, not moving and looked up at me, uncertainty reflected in her eyes.

I assured her that it was okay not to help, and bent over holding her close.

Jake knelt down on the cold, damp ground and took the container from his grandfather. He placed it gently in the hole and then stood up, the deep blue eyes of his father solemnly fixed on Grandpa Jack, who grasped him in a fierce hug.

Mark's brother, Dick took a small spade and squatting down filled the hole with the clotted earth, tamping it down. No one spoke. Just the wind and the music.

Finally, Jack offered a silent prayer and then announced we'd meet at a local restaurant.

I encircled the children and to avoid any controversy, waited until Ann's family had gone. Once released, Lucy and Jake went on ahead scampering on the heels of their cousins.

Alone, I stood and gazed up at the cloudy sky and knew Mark was finally at peace. It was damned cold, even for March. And it was beginning to sleet. My coat pulled tight, I tucked my head down against the biting wind and made my way slowly down the cobbled hill.

The End: Late That Summer

Stretched out in the calm eddy, my toes dug down under the wet sand, I lifted my face to the waning summer sun. Down the beach in the shimmer of the late afternoon, I could see the silhouettes of the children and hear their laughter blending in with the repetitive refrain of the waves when they rolled in to the shore.

It was here where I'd been before the world shifted, the recollections rushing back. When I closed my eyes, I could hear the lilting timbre of Mark's voice as he tacked into the wind bringing the swift catamaran about. His deep laugh when I plummeted off and shrieked at him that he did it on purpose. He hauled me back in the boat, and we made love on the tarp while the sky and water merged and faded into that crimson you only get on the southern Gulf.

My memories are no longer harsh. The postscript of Mark's life is the goodness that survives in his children. After all, no one can really plan a life. We have little control. Our limited brains can do so much and our weak hearts get lost in the shuffle of life's deck.

I opened my eyes when I heard the kids splashing towards me.

Lucy was hungry. Jake taunted her thrusting a wriggling crab in her face, telling her to eat this!

"Yuck, get that away from me! Mom! Make him stop." Lucy yelped running into the water, Jake fast on her heels.

Grinning, I hollered out at them and stood up. It was almost time for supper.

"Five more minutes," Jake pleaded.

"Nope. Zero more minutes. I'll race you both!"

Jake dashed ahead and left Lucy and me woefully behind as I paused to stop and catch my breath.

Lucy caught my hand.

I grinned. "Do you know who I love the most in the whole wide world?"

"Me." She smiled back and then added, "And Jake too, even though he's second."

Epilogue

Over 25 years have passed since my husband died. When I tell the story about what happened to my family, it seems almost unreal, like it happened to someone else or is a made-up movie event. The friends who lived it with me serve as reminders that it was real, and I'm forever grateful for them, then and now. Some folks, never reconnected with me, and I'm as much to blame, since I didn't try hard to make it right. At the time, I could only do so much, and the deluge is under the damn, so to speak. Many, in both families, are gone and those who remain, stay connected, thanks to the Facebook miracle and savvy young adults.

My children are grown and probably bear some scars, as I do, but seem to be happy, content young people who've done well and continue to amaze me with their passion, smarts and humor. It's grand to really like your 'kids'. I never remarried. Somehow, I knew that I could raise my children and that they needed me completely (and we benefitted from good therapy). I can't take all the credit for the amazing people they turned out to be. They were mentored by a grandfather, who grew up in the Jim Crow south and infuriated their grandmother because he wouldn't leave a restaurant in rural Georgia when a busload of black folks sat down, during the early 60's. She fumed, outside in the hot car, while my daddy and I ate lunch. The drive home was mighty long.

At my dad's funeral, he was 93, both my kids spoke and shared their experiences of a life with him as an anchor (my mom died early at 72). My dad once said that maybe the good Lord knew that Mark wouldn't have been the daddy they needed. And I've got to say, I don't know diddly squat, in comparison to the good Lord. My daughter, Lucy, the old soul in the family, declares it was all meant to be.

Sam went on to do what he should have done at his age; marry, have kids and I figure he's a great father. We keep in touch. In some way, he saved me; maybe, I saved him too,

Over the years, the science and fears about HIV/AIDS have changed. The fear folks lived with, not just the horrible death and dying, but the need to cover it up was tangible. Even now, after all this time, when people ask me how my husband died, I don't tell them AIDS right away, I wait, and if I figure I'm going to really know them, I share it later when we establish a relationship.

I first heard about the science and the 'Plague' genetic connection, after Mark had gone, probably, 1993 or so. A close friend, who was working with HIV folks mentioned genetic trials and suggested I might get involved. I declined, but thought it interesting. Years later, I found myself hearing about the genetic link again, this time, with more certainty. While I have no idea if I am genetically immune, my fore bearers are English and Scots; the 'ancestors protecting me' comment from Hazel, the medium in Casadega never far from mind.

Acknowledgements

First, an enormous thank you to Janice Shay, literary agent extraordinaire, who had the vision and encouragement that helped me see this through. Y'all, she rocks!

It is difficult to know where to begin because I am so grateful to many, a number of whom are in the book (Some people requested I not use their real names nor did I use my husband's last name.): Marsha; Annie; Jeffrey; Sears; Alicia; Christine; Mike and Ruth; Warren and Karen, who is gone; Hal; Loren; Alan; Kate; Dick; the St. Edward's church folks; and the NKOTB, for their care of my daughter and concern for my husband. Philip, (Mark's brother) and his dad have passed on, as have my parents.

My writing group buddies and the Book Club in Auburn were always there for support and honest critique even across the distance.

Then, those close friends, not specifically named, who heard, listened and offered housing, food, a shoulder to cry on and whatever, whenever: Janice and Mark; Drew; Johnny M.; Marsha J. and Nancy; Russ and Diane; the Savannah group, Millie, Sherry and Dr. John; nieces and nephews, the college community. Any I've missed, it is because I'm old and addled.

And finally, how lucky to have my grown-up children, Lucy and Jake, who when asked about telling this story reminded me that 'it's what happened a long time ago, Mom'.

In closing, I want to acknowledge those we lost from AIDS during this time. They were many and should never be dismissed or forgotten.

Note from the Author

Word-of-mouth is crucial for any author to succeed. If you enjoyed *A Red Door*, please leave a review online—anywhere you are able. Even if it's just a sentence or two. It would make all the difference and would be very much appreciated.

Thanks!
Kathryn

Thank you so much for reading one of our **Biography / Memoirs**.

If you enjoyed our book, please check out our recommendation for your next great read!

Z.O.S. by Kay Merkel Boruff

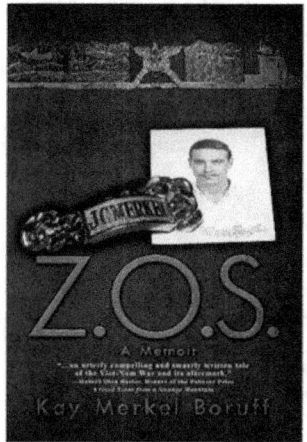

"...dazzling in its specificity and intensity."

–C.W. Smith, author of *Understanding Women*

View other Black Rose Writing titles at www.blackrosewriting.com/books and use promo code **PRINT** to receive a **20% discount** when purchasing.

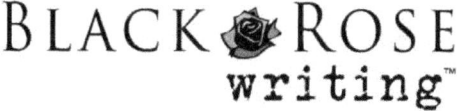

www.ingramcontent.com/pod-product-compliance
Lightning Source LLC
Chambersburg PA
CBHW071422080526
44587CB00014B/1721